Introduction to Cardiopulm
Exercise Testi

Introduction to Cardiopulmonary Exercise Testing

Andrew M. Luks, MD
University of Washington School of Medicine,
Seattle, WA, USA

Robb W. Glenny, MD
University of Washington School of Medicine,
Seattle, WA, USA

H. Thomas Robertson, MD
University of Washington School of Medicine,
Seattle, WA, USA

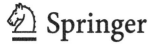 Springer

Andrew M. Luks, MD
University of Washington School of Medicine
Seattle, WA, USA

Robb W. Glenny, MD
University of Washington School of Medicine
Seattle, WA, USA

H. Thomas Robertson, MD
University of Washington School of Medicine
Seattle, WA, USA

ISBN 978-1-4614-6282-8   ISBN 978-1-4614-6283-5 (eBook)
DOI 10.1007/978-1-4614-6283-5
Springer New York Heidelberg Dordrecht London

Library of Congress Control Number: 2013930552

Printed on acid-free paper

Springer is part of Springer Science+Business Media (www.springer.com)

Acknowledgements

The authors would like to thank John Smith, the lead technologist in our exercise laboratory, for his assistance in collecting data for inclusion in the cases in this primer and, most importantly, for his diligence and dedication in keeping our cardiopulmonary exercise testing program running as well as it has for many years.

The authors would also like to thank Brownie Schoene, Bruce Culver, Erik Swenson, and other faculty and fellows who have regularly attended our weekly exercise conference since its inception over 30 years ago and helped make it one of the most stimulating parts of our week.

Contents

Chapter 1
Introduction to the Primer

Keywords Adenosine triphosphate (ATP) • Cardiomyopathy • Cardiopulmonary exercise test • Chronic obstructive pulmonary disease (COPD) • Exercise limitation

EXERCISE: A MULTISYSTEM PROCESS

Most activities of daily living, such as rising from a chair, opening a jar, lifting a box, or walking at a slow pace, require only a modest amount of muscle strength or endurance, and do not involve significant demands on the respiratory or cardiovascular systems. However, vigorous aerobic exercises, such as running or sustained stair climbing, require tight integration of multiple systems in the body including the respiratory, cardiovascular, and neuromuscular systems (Fig. 1.1).

Each of these systems has important functions. The respiratory system, for example, is a ventilatory pump, moving oxygen from the atmosphere to the alveoli and carbon dioxide from the alveoli to the atmosphere. It must also provide an effective means of exchanging oxygen and carbon dioxide across the thin alveolar walls. The heart is responsible for pumping oxygenated blood to the exercising muscles as well as returning oxygen-poor and carbon dioxide-rich blood to the gas-exchanging surfaces of the lungs. Finally, the nervous system must transmit signals to the exercising muscles through upper and lower motor neurons while the muscles must extract oxygen from the blood, generate adenosine triphosphate (ATP) in the mitochondria, and contract with force sufficient to support the intended activity.

The systems do not work independently but rather in a highly coordinated manner. The most significant interdependence is the delivery

A.M. Luks et al., *Introduction to Cardiopulmonary Exercise Testing*, DOI 10.1007/978-1-4614-6283-5_1, © Springer Science+Business Media New York 2013

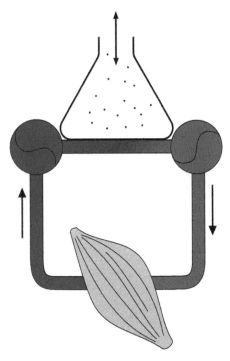

Fig. 1.1 Multiple systems including the lungs at *top*, *right*, and *left* side of the heart, denoted in *blue* and *red*, respectively, and the neuromuscular system work together to generate sustained high-level exercise. Problems in one or several of these systems can lead to diminished exercise capacity

of oxygen to the working muscles. The lungs must efficiently oxygenate blood returning from the venous system, and the left heart must then distribute this oxygenated blood to skeletal, cardiac, and respiratory muscles in proportion to the amount of work being done by the individual muscles. All of this coordination must occur in proportion to the amount of work being performed, whether it is mild, moderate, or extreme exercise.

Pathology in any of the important systems noted above can lead to limitations in an individual's exercise tolerance. In patients with cardiomyopathy, for example, delivery of oxygen to the exercising muscles is insufficient to support mitochondrial ATP generation and, as a result, muscle contraction. Similarly, in patients with severe chronic obstructive pulmonary disease (COPD), altered respiratory system mechanics impair ventilation and the patient cannot eliminate carbon dioxide (CO_2) being produced in the exercising muscles. Rising CO_2, in turn, causes progressive dyspnea, which forces the patient to cease exercising. In some cases, failure within a single system leads to exercise limitation, while in other situations multiple systems are deficient at the same time.

EVALUATING EXERCISE CAPACITY: THE CARDIOPULMONARY EXERCISE TEST

Patients often discount the importance of loss of exercise tolerance as a significant symptom, when in reality diminished exercise tolerance is a sensitive marker of underlying disease in the respiratory, cardiac, or neuromuscular systems. When patients present with this symptom, comprehensive evaluation including history and physical examination and basic laboratory and other studies such as chest radiography and pulmonary function testing are warranted to help determine the etiology of the problem. In many cases, these limited steps are sufficient to arrive at an answer but in other cases, the source of the problem remains unexplained and further evaluation is necessary.

One of the studies that can be used to determine the etiology of unexplained dyspnea on exertion is the cardiopulmonary exercise test (CPET). This test requires 20–30 minutes to perform using either a treadmill or a cycle ergometer, during which time the patient's heart rate, oxygen saturation, and electrocardiogram (ECG) are monitored continuously, while blood pressure is measured intermittently. The individual wears a tight fitting mask to allow collection of all exhaled gases to measure minute ventilation, oxygen uptake, and carbon dioxide production. In some cases, blood gases are also measured using a radial artery catheter or intermittent arterial punctures. The test is far more comprehensive than the standard exercise treadmill test and provides a wealth of information that can be used to help identify which of the major systems is primarily responsible for the limited exercise capacity.

Cardiopulmonary exercise testing can help determine the system that is limiting exercise by demonstrating characteristic alterations in the normal physiologic responses to exercise. Patients with cardiac disease, for example, manifest physiologic responses that provide evidence of impaired oxygen delivery to the exercising muscles while patients with very severe COPD show evidence of impaired ventilatory capacity as the major limiting factor. These altered physiologic responses present as characteristic patterns of data on cardiopulmonary exercise testing. Careful analysis of the data to identify these patterns can potentially illuminate why the patient's exercise capacity is impaired.

Beyond identifying the source of exercise limitation, this testing modality has a variety of other uses in clinical medicine including assessing fitness for surgery, monitoring disease progression, and evaluating responses to treatment. It may also be used as part of research protocols or training and assessment programs in highly conditioned athletes.

THE ROLE OF THIS PRIMER

While the data generated in cardiopulmonary exercise tests is useful for addressing the issues described above, the volume of data can be overwhelming to those just developing their skills in test implementation and interpretation. It can be difficult to identify the characteristic patterns in various disease states and avoid certain pitfalls in the test interpretation process. This primer is intended to minimize this complexity and provide an introduction to clinical cardiopulmonary exercise testing. Designed for both first-time users and practitioners looking to refresh their knowledge, the primer is meant to provide immediate easy access to the necessary information to use these tests in clinical practice.

The primary goal of the primer is to present the reader with an approach to interpreting testing data and identifying the primary system limiting exercise capacity. Rather than focusing on decision algorithms, our approach relies more on the ability to recognize patterns in the data and weigh the relative importance of various factors. The pattern recognition approach we describe is simplest when there is a single affected system, but it is important to recognize that patients often present for testing with multiple organ system abnormalities that impair their overall exercise performance. Our focus throughout this primer will be to identify the primary system limiting exercise by observing characteristic alterations in the normal physiologic responses to exercise.

The reader will complete this primer with a firm understanding of the normal physiologic responses to exercise, how those responses change in various disease states, how to conduct a CPET, and how to interpret the acquired data to determine which organ system is limiting exercise in a given patient.

ORGANIZATION OF THE PRIMER

Because some of the language of exercise testing is not part of a general medical knowledge base, we begin with a "Glossary of Terms" (Chap. 2) used in the conduct and interpretation of exercise tests. The glossary is followed by a chapter entitled "Cardiac and Respiratory Responses to Exercise in Health and Disease" (Chap. 3), which provides an overview of the physiologic responses to exercise in normal individuals and those with different categories of disease. The chapter "Conducting a Cardiopulmonary Exercise Test" (Chap. 4) describes procedures to follow before, during, and after the test to insure patient safety and appropriate data collection. Finally the section "Interpreting the Results of the Cardiopulmonary Exercise Test" (Chap. 5) takes you through the steps of interpreting and documenting the test results, including approaches to identify an essential finding for interpretation of the test results, the ventilatory threshold. The final two sections of the primer include resources to improve your test interpretation skills. The "Sample Cases" (Chap. 6) section includes known cases that demonstrate the basic patterns of exercise limitation you are likely to encounter. This section is followed by the "Self-Assessment Cases" chapter (Chap. 7), which provides an opportunity for you to work through and interpret data from a series of patients and identify the cause of exercise limitation.

The physiology underlying exercise and cardiopulmonary exercise testing can be complex. We have deliberately simplified the material in this primer in order to make it more accessible to individuals new to or rediscovering this testing modality and make it possible to master the basics in a short period of time. However, the primer is only an introduction to the testing modality and those learners interested in acquiring detailed information about the underlying physiology of exercise and CPET interpretation are encouraged to explore the more extensive resources cited below.

ADDITIONAL RESOURCES

American Thoracic Society/American College of Chest Physicians. ATS/ACCP statement on cardiopulmonary exercise testing. Am J Respir Crit Care Med. 2003;167:211–77.

Balady G, Arena R, Sietsema KE, Myers J, Coke L, Fletcher GF, Forman DE, Franklin B, Guazzi M, Gulati M, Keteyian SJ, Lavie CJ, Macko R, Mancini D, Milani RV. American Heart Association scientific statement: a clinician's guide to cardiopulmonary exercise testing in adults. Circulation. 2010;122:191–225.

Jones NL. Clinical exercise testing. 4th ed. Philadelphia: Saunders; 1997.

Wasserman K, Hansen JE, Sue DY, Stringer WW, Whipp BJ. Principles of exercise testing and interpretation. 4th ed. Philadelphia: Lippincott, Williams and Wilkins; 2005.

Chapter 2
Glossary of Terms

Keywords Alveolar-arterial oxygen difference • Alveolar carbon dioxide • Alveolar oxygen • Anaerobic threshold • Carbon dioxide output • Cardiac output • Dead space fraction • End-tidal carbon dioxide • End-tidal oxygen • Forced expiratory volume in one second • Forced vital capacity • Heart rate reserve • Lactate threshold • Maximum oxygen consumption • Maximum voluntary ventilation • Minute ventilation • Oxygen consumption • Oxygen content • Oxygen pulse (O_2 pulse) • Oxygen saturation • Power • Progressive work exercise test • Respiratory exchange ratio • Respiratory quotient • Spirometry • Tidal volume • Ventilation • Ventilatory equivalents for carbon dioxide • Ventilatory equivalents for oxygen • Ventilatory reserve • Ventilatory threshold

The following list contains terms with which you will need to be familiar for the conduct and interpretation of cardiopulmonary exercise tests. Definitions of the terms are provided here, while Fig. 2.1 provides a visual description of where the values of these parameters are determined in the integrated exercise system described in Chap. 1. Detailed descriptions of the expected changes in these parameters during exercise in healthy people and those with underlying disease are provided in Chap. 3.

- *Alveolar–arterial oxygen difference* $(A-a)\Delta O_2$ is the difference between the alveolar and arterial partial pressures of oxygen. The arterial value is determined by arterial blood gas while the alveolar values are calculated using the alveolar gas equation and the partial pressure of carbon dioxide measured by arterial blood gas. The units are mmHg.

- *Carbon dioxide output* ($\dot{V}CO_2$) refers to the amount of carbon dioxide (CO_2) exhaled from the body per unit time. It is

A.M. Luks et al., *Introduction to Cardiopulmonary Exercise Testing*, DOI 10.1007/978-1-4614-6283-5_2,

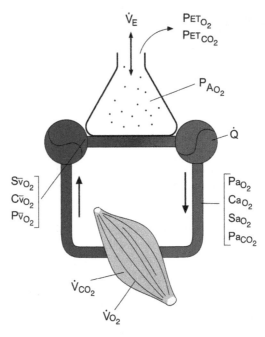

Fig. 2.1 A visual description of the location in the integrated exercise system at which the values of many of the parameters obtained during cardiopulmonary exercise testing are obtained. The red structures refer to the left side of the heart and the arterial circulation while the blue structures refer to the venous circulation and the right side of the heart. The pulmonary circulation is denoted by the horizontal segment with a color gradient connecting the right and left heart

expressed in ml/minute. Note that carbon dioxide output is measured at the mouth and can differ from carbon dioxide *production* at the tissue level but in the steady state, production and output are the same.

- *Cardiac output* ($\dot{Q}$) refers to the amount of blood pumped out of the left side of the heart each minute. The units are liters/minutes. Direct measurement requires placement of a pulmonary artery catheter but alternative assessments of this parameter can be obtained using the measured oxygen consumption (described further in Chap. 3).
- *Dead-space fraction* (V_D/V_T) is a measure of the physiologic dead space of the lungs and represents the fraction of inspired air that does not exchange gas with capillary blood. It has no

units, as it is expressed as a fraction of the same units. This value can be calculated if arterial blood gas values are obtained. Some cardiopulmonary exercise test systems provide an estimate of the dead-space fraction based on end-tidal carbon dioxide measurements but these values are poor surrogates for the more accurate measurements derived from blood gases and should not be used to calculate a dead-space fraction.

- *End-tidal partial pressure of carbon dioxide* ($\text{P\textsc{et}CO}_2$) is the partial pressure of carbon dioxide in the exhaled gas at the end of exhalation. The units are mmHg. It is a surrogate for alveolar carbon dioxide tensions (PaCO_2).
- *End-tidal partial pressure of oxygen* ($\text{P\textsc{et}O}_2$) refers to the partial pressure of oxygen in exhaled gas at the end of exhalation. Its units are mmHg. It is a surrogate for alveolar oxygen tensions (PaO_2).
- *Forced expiratory volume in one second* (FEV_1) is the volume of air exhaled in the first second of a forced vital capacity maneuver. It is measured using spirometry and its units are liters. The value is often expressed in terms of the percent predicted for the test subject given their gender, age, and height. It can be used to help estimate the maximum voluntary ventilation (*see* below) and to assess the test subject's pulmonary function.
- *Forced vital capacity* (FVC) is the volume of air exhaled in a forced exhalation from total lung capacity. It is measured using spirometry and its units are liters. The value is often expressed in terms of the percent predicted for the test subject given their gender, age, and height and is used as part of the assessment of the test subject's pulmonary function.
- *FEV₁/FVC ratio* is the ratio of the two spirometry parameters described above. Because the parameters that comprise the ratio have the same units (liters), the ratio is a unit-less measurement. The ratio is used to help identify abnormal lung function with low values being consistent with obstructive lung disease.
- *Heart rate reserve* refers to the difference between the maximum heart rate reached by the subject at peak exercise and the average value for age-predicted maximum (220 – age). The reader should be aware that cardiologists sometimes use the same phrase to refer to the difference between the resting heart rate and the maximum heart rate achieved during an exercise treadmill test. Throughout this primer, we will use the former definition of the term. As will be described later in the primer, the problem with application of this calculation to test interpretation

is that there is substantial variability in the maximum heart rate in normal subjects of similar age.

■ *Maximum voluntary ventilation* (MVV) refers to the maximum level of ventilation that can be generated by the subject per minute. Patients are instructed to take maximum breaths in and out of a spirometer, as fast as they can, for 12 s. The ventilation achieved during this period is multiplied by 5 to give an estimate of the MVV. This value can also be estimated by taking the forced expiratory volume in one second (FEV_1) measured by spirometry and multiplying this value by 40 [1, 2].

■ *Minute ventilation* ($\dot{V}E$) refers to the volume of air exhaled in 1 minute. The units of this parameter, which is measured at the mouth, are liters/minutes.

■ *Oxygen consumption* ($\dot{V}O_2$) refers to oxygen uptake from the lung each minute, as measured at the mouth. The units are ml/minute. *Maximum oxygen consumption* ($\dot{V}O_{2\max}$) is the amount of oxygen being consumed at peak exercise (i.e., at the point that the person cannot do any more and has to stop exercising). It is measured in the same units as oxygen consumption but is often normalized for the subject's weight in kilograms in which case the units are ml/kg/minute.

■ *Oxygen content* refers to the amount of oxygen being carried in the blood bound to hemoglobin or dissolved in plasma. It is a function of the hemoglobin concentration, hemoglobin oxygen saturation, and partial pressure of oxygen. The units are ml O_2/100 ml blood. When measured in the arterial circulation, it is denoted CaO_2, while when measured in the venous circulation it is denoted CvO_2. Values obtained from blood in the pulmonary arterial circulation are referred to as the mixed venous oxygen content and are denoted $C\overline{v}O_2$.

■ *Oxygen pulse or O_2 pulse* refers to the volume of oxygen consumed per heartbeat. It is calculated by dividing the oxygen consumption ($\dot{V}O_2$) by the simultaneously measured heart rate per minute. The units are ml O_2/beat. The parameter is used as a surrogate measure for an individual's stroke volume at end-exercise and is described in greater detail in Chap. 3.

■ *Oxygen saturation* refers to the percentage of hemoglobin binding sites that are occupied by oxygen at a given time. When measured in the arterial circulation, it is denoted SaO_2, while when measured in the venous circulation it is denoted SvO_2. Values obtained from blood in the pulmonary arterial circulation are referred to as the mixed venous oxygen saturation and are denoted $S\overline{v}O_2$.

- *Power* is work per unit time. In an exercise test utilizing a cycle ergometer, the power output can be measured precisely and is expressed in watts. For exercise tests using a treadmill there are equations incorporating the speed and grade of the treadmill and the subject's weight to estimate power output, but those estimates are not fully reliable.

- *Progressive work exercise test*: In most cardiopulmonary exercise tests, the subjects are asked to walk/run at steadily increasing speed and grade or pedal against increasing resistance. The rate at which those factors are increased is referred to as the *"ramp"* and indicates how much the power output will increase per minute during the test. In certain situations, constant work-rate tests are performed in which the treadmill speed/grade or bicycle resistance does not change.

- *Respiratory exchange ratio* (R) refers to the ratio of carbon dioxide output to oxygen uptake $(\dot{V}CO_2/\dot{V}O_2)$ measured at the mouth. In the steady state, this value is the same as the *respiratory quotient* (*RQ*), the ratio of carbon dioxide production to oxygen consumption $(\dot{V}CO_2/\dot{V}O_2)$ measured at the tissue level. *The respiratory exchange ratio* is influenced both by the metabolically determined RQ and by the transient hyperventilation that is a normal feature of a maximum exercise effort.

- *Tidal volume* (VT) refers to the volume of a single breath. It is measured at the mouth and the units are liters.

- *Ventilatory equivalents for carbon dioxide* $(\dot{V}E/\dot{V}CO_2)$ refers to the number of liters of ventilation per liter of carbon dioxide output. It is used as a marker of the efficiency of ventilation with abnormally high values occurring due to hyperventilation or increased dead space. Because $\dot{V}E$ and $\dot{V}CO_2$ both have the same units (liters/minutes), the term $\dot{V}E/\dot{V}CO_2$ has no units.

- *Ventilatory equivalents for oxygen* $(\dot{V}E/\dot{V}O_2)$ refers to the number of liters of ventilation per liter of oxygen consumed. It is used as a marker of the efficiency of ventilation with abnormally high values occurring due to hyperventilation or increased dead space. Because $\dot{V}E$ and $\dot{V}O_2$ both have the same units (liters/minutes), the term $\dot{V}E/\dot{V}O_2$ has no units.

- *Ventilatory reserve* is also referred to as the "breathing reserve" and refers to the difference between the maximum minute ventilation reached by the subject at peak exercise and their maximum voluntary ventilation. In some cases, the value of the $FEV_1 \times 40$ is substituted for the maximum voluntary ventilation in this determination.

- *Ventilatory threshold* refers to an important point in a cardio-pulmonary exercise test where a number of ventilatory parameters exhibit a threshold-like response during progressive exercise. It is temporally related to the development of a lactic acidosis. Other terms for this transition timepoint include *"lactate threshold"* or *"anaerobic threshold."* Identifying whether this threshold is present is a critical part of test interpretation and is discussed in greater detail in the chapter on interpreting cardiopulmonary exercise tests (Chap. 5).

REFERENCES

1. Hansen JE, Sue DY, Wasserman K. Predicted values for clinical exercise testing. Am Rev Respir Dis. 1984;129(suppl):S49–55.
2. Campbell SC. A comparison of the maximum volume ventilation with forced expiratory volume in one second: an assessment of subject cooperation. J Occup Med. 1982;24:531–3.

Chapter 3
Cardiac and Respiratory Responses to Exercise in Health and Disease

Keywords Arteriovenous oxygen content difference • Arterial oxygen content • Blood pressure • Cardiac limitation • Diastolic dysfunction • Fick equation • Heart rate • Hemoglobin • Ideal body weight • Idiopathic pulmonary fibrosis • Interstitial lung disease • Mitochondria • Mitochondrial myopathy • Mixed venous oxygen content • Neuromuscular disease • Partial pressure of oxygen • Partial pressure of carbon dioxide • Peripheral vascular disease • pH • Pulmonary artery pressure • Pulmonary vascular disease • Stroke volume • Venous oxygen content • Ventilatory limitation

INTRODUCTION

Appropriate interpretation of cardiopulmonary exercise tests depends on an understanding of exercise physiology. The focus of this chapter is the expected physiologic responses to exercise in normal individuals and how the physiologic responses deviate from the expected patterns in various disease states. We begin by describing a key parameter that is used to assess overall exercise capacity, maximum oxygen consumption, and discuss its relationship to maximum cardiac function. We then review the expected physiologic responses to exercise in normal individuals and, finally, examine the pattern of physiologic responses expected in disorders causing exercise limitation.

A.M. Luks et al., *Introduction to Cardiopulmonary Exercise Testing*, DOI 10.1007/978-1-4614-6283-5_3, © Springer Science+Business Media New York 2013

ASSESSING OVERALL EXERCISE CAPACITY: MAXIMUM OXYGEN CONSUMPTION

As described in Chap. 1, the ability to perform sustained, vigorous exercise depends on the participation of multiple systems including the respiratory, cardiovascular, and neuromuscular systems. In particular, several important tasks must be accomplished by these and other systems to support physical activity, including:

- Ventilation to deliver oxygen to the alveoli and eliminate carbon dioxide.
- Gas exchange to move oxygen from the alveoli to the blood and carbon dioxide from the blood to the alveoli.
- Maintenance of hemoglobin stores to bind and carry oxygen to the tissues.
- Delivery of oxygenated blood to the exercising tissues and carbon dioxide to the lungs.
- Extraction of oxygen by the muscle mitochondria where ATP is generated to support muscle contraction.

To assess an individual's capacity to perform all of these tasks and conduct sustained, vigorous exercise, one of the most useful parameters is the maximum oxygen consumption or $\dot{V}O_{2\max}$. Oxygen consumption ($\dot{V}O_2$) describes how much oxygen is being used by the tissues per minute, while maximum oxygen consumption ($\dot{V}O_{2\max}$) is the amount of oxygen being used at peak exercise (i.e., right at the point that the person cannot do any more and has to stop exercising).

To understand the value of this parameter in assessing overall exercise capacity, we can look at the determinants of $\dot{V}O_2$ using the Fick equation:

$$\dot{Q} = \frac{\dot{V}O_2}{CaO_2 - C\bar{v}O_2}, \tag{3.1}$$

where

$\dot{Q}$ = cardiac output, CaO_2 = arterial oxygen content,   and $C\bar{v}O_2$ = mixed venous oxygen content.

Rearranging this equation we see that

$$\dot{V}O_2 = \dot{Q} \times (CaO_2 - C\bar{v}O_2) \tag{3.2}$$

This tells us that oxygen consumption is a function of cardiac output and the arteriovenous oxygen content difference.

Recall that

$$CaO_2 = [(1.39 \times Hb \times SaO_2) + (0.003 \times PaO_2)] \quad (3.3)$$

and

$$C\overline{v}O_2 = [(1.39 \times Hb \times S\overline{v}O_2) + (0.003 \times P\overline{v}O_2)], \quad (3.4)$$

where Hb = hemoglobin concentration, PaO_2 = partial pressure of oxygen in arterial blood, $P\overline{v}O_2$ = partial pressure of oxygen in mixed venous blood, SaO_2 = arterial oxygen saturation, and $S\overline{v}O_2$ = mixed venous oxygen saturation.

Oxygen consumption is therefore dependent on the hemoglobin concentration, the arterial partial pressure and saturation of oxygen (reflecting the adequacy of the ventilatory pump and gas exchange), and the mixed venous saturation and partial pressure of oxygen (reflecting the ability of the tissues to extract and utilize oxygen). As a result, $\dot{V}O_{2\,max}$ gives us information about many of the systems that are necessary to generate sustained, vigorous exercise; the higher the $\dot{V}O_{2\,max}$, the more effective all of these systems are at performing their tasks and the greater the person's exercise capacity.

Maximum oxygen consumption can be expressed in absolute terms (ml O_2 consumed per minute) or it can be normalized for the person's body weight (ml O_2 consumed per minute per kg of body weight). While the convention has been to use the weight-normalized measurement, based on earlier studies with athletes and young normal subjects, the current obesity epidemic now makes ml/(kg actual weight)/minute a less appropriate adjustment for many subjects, and a more meaningful adjustment now is to use predictive equations that incorporate height adjustment rather than weight adjustment. With these equations we compare the $\dot{V}O_{2\,max}$ relative to that expected for a person of the same gender, age, and height and express it in terms of the percent predicted for that individual. This is conceptually equivalent to normalizing the maximum oxygen consumption to ideal body weight.

Maximum oxygen consumption will vary from individual to individual. Whereas the $\dot{V}O_{2\,max}$ for an average 30-year-old person might be 35–40 ml/kg/minute, an elite cyclist or cross-country skier might have a $\dot{V}O_{2\,max}$ of 85 ml/kg/minute. Patients with a cardiomyopathy, on the other hand, may have a $\dot{V}O_{2\,max}$ as low as 15 ml/kg/minute or less, severely limiting the capacity to perform normal activities of daily living. Maximum oxygen consumption declines with age, although that decline may be substantially delayed in physically active subjects.

ASSESSING CARDIAC FUNCTION: CARDIAC OUTPUT AND STROKE VOLUME

When evaluating an individual's exercise capacity, a considerable amount of attention is given to the adequacy of their cardiac function. In particular, it is useful to have information about the cardiac output as well as the stroke volume. Measuring these parameters directly requires placement of a pulmonary artery catheter, an invasive step that is typically not done in most exercise studies. While noninvasive methods that rely on the inert gas technique are increasingly being used for this purpose in clinical practice, in most cases we can use the measurements of $\dot{V}O_2$ and $\dot{V}O_{2\,max}$ to provide information about these parameters.

CARDIAC OUTPUT

To understand how the patient's $\dot{V}O_{2\,max}$ provides information about the patient's cardiac output, we can refer back to the Fick equation above (3.1). It turns out that for both normal subjects and patients with cardiac disease, about 80% of the oxygen will be extracted from arterial blood with a maximum effort. In other words, the arterio-venous oxygen content difference ($CaO_2 - C\overline{v}O_2$) is largely the same across both normal individuals and patients with cardiac disease at maximum exercise. As a result, the wide range of $\dot{V}O_{2\,max}$ measurements observed among healthy normal individuals and patients with cardiac impairment are determined primarily by the wide range of maximum cardiac outputs. It is for this reason that for either normal subjects or patients with cardiac disease, we can conclude that the higher the patient's $\dot{V}O_{2\,max}$, the higher their cardiac output and vice versa. The $\dot{V}O_{2\,max}$ is not giving us a quantitative measure of the cardiac output itself, but is ordinarily directly proportional to that measurement. However, if significant anemia is present, the $\dot{V}O_{2\,max}$ will be low relative to the actual cardiac output.

STROKE VOLUME

Oxygen consumption at maximum exercise can also be used to estimate stroke volume. To understand this, we can return to (3.2) above. Because cardiac output is a function of heart rate and stroke volume, we can express this relationship in the following manner:

$$\dot{V}O_2 = HR \times SV \times (CaO_2 - C\overline{v}O_2), \qquad (3.5)$$

where HR is heart rate and SV is stroke volume.

Rearranging this, we get the following:

$$\frac{\dot{V}O_2}{HR} = SV \times (CaO_2 - C\bar{v}O_2) \tag{3.6}$$

The term $\dot{V}O_2 / HR$ is referred to as the O_2 pulse and represents the amount of oxygen consumed per heartbeat.

We can see from (3.6) that the O_2 pulse increases with exercise due to a modest early increase in stroke volume and a substantial increase in the arteriovenous oxygen content difference (from about 5 ml O_2/100 ml blood at rest to 15 ml O_2/100 ml blood at maximum exercise). At maximum exercise the arteriovenous oxygen content difference stops increasing. Because the arteriovenous oxygen content difference is about 15 ml O_2/100 ml blood at end-exercise, both in normal individuals and those with cardiac disease, the O_2 pulse serves as a good surrogate of stroke volume, provided the hemoglobin content is normal.

The O_2 pulse should increase progressively with exercise, reflecting both the normal increase in stroke volume at the initiation of exercise and the progressive increase in the arteriovenous content difference with increasing work. Hence an early plateau in O_2 pulse or even a late decrease in O_2 pulse with increasing oxygen consumption is a helpful sign suggesting an exercise-associated decrease in stroke volume, as is observed in patients with diastolic dysfunction.

EXERCISE RESPONSES IN NORMAL INDIVIDUALS

While $\dot{V}O_{2\,max}$, cardiac output, and stroke volume are important variables in assessing exercise capacity, there are a variety of other parameters that can be monitored during a progressive work exercise test to yield information about an individual's exercise capacity. As the power output increases during a cardiopulmonary exercise test, these parameters change in a predictable manner, which defines the exercise response in normal individuals. The expected changes for these parameters, which were defined in Chap. 2, are described below with the parameters being listed in alphabetical order.

As you read these descriptions of the expected changes with each parameter you will notice that a key point in the time course of many of these parameters is what is referred to as the "ventilatory threshold."

This term refers to an important point in a cardiopulmonary exercise test where a number of ventilatory parameters exhibit a threshold-like response during progressive exercise. Other terms for this transition, which is temporally related to the development of a lactic acidosis, include "lactate threshold" or "anaerobic threshold," but at our institution we prefer to use the term "ventilatory threshold." While there is debate on the functional significance of the events in muscle leading to the lactic acidosis, there is agreement that the ventilatory threshold identifies a level of exertion where lactate spills out of the exercising muscles into the circulation. The ventilatory threshold and how it is identified during a cardiopulmonary exercise test are described in much greater detail in Chap. 5.

In a cardiopulmonary exercise test report, many of the variables described below are presented in both tabular and graphical format. Traditionally, the graphical data presentation is the "9-Box plot," a format created by Karlman Wasserman and his colleagues, in which the key variables are displayed in nine separate graphs on the same page [1]. By convention, the graphs are always displayed in the same order within this plot. The characteristic changes for many of the variables described below are presented in this 9-Box plot format in Fig. 3.1.

ARTERIAL PARTIAL PRESSURE OF CARBON DIOXIDE ($PaCO_2$)

The $PaCO_2$ reflects a balance between how much carbon dioxide is produced in the tissues on the one hand and eliminated in the lungs by alveolar ventilation on the other. This parameter remains relatively constant during exercise until the ventilatory threshold is reached because alveolar ventilation increases at a rate proportional to the increasing quantities of carbon dioxide being produced in the tissue. Once the ventilatory threshold occurs, the developing metabolic acidosis triggers an increase in minute ventilation such that minute ventilation and alveolar ventilation now rise at a greater rate than carbon dioxide production. As a result, there is a drop in the $PaCO_2$. Because arterial blood gases are not collected in all cardiopulmonary exercise tests, the *end-tidal carbon dioxide tension* ($PetCO_2$) is used as a surrogate measure for the $PaCO_2$. It is expected to change in the same direction as the $PaCO_2$, although there will be small absolute differences between the parameters that are more marked in patients with underlying lung disease (Fig. 3.1i).

ARTERIAL PARTIAL PRESSURE OF OXYGEN (PaO_2)

This parameter remains relatively constant throughout exercise, although a small subset of elite aerobic athletes may show a decrease

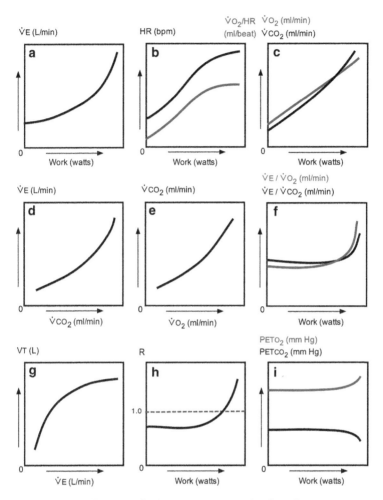

Fig. 3.1 Expected changes for key parameters in the physiologic response to exercise displayed in the 9-Box plot format commonly used in cardiopulmonary exercise testing. Labels for the y-axis variables are presented on the top of each graph due to space considerations. Note that for the variables on the x- and y-axes the lowest values are in the *lower left-hand corner* of each plot. The *arrows* denote the direction of increasing values for both variables

in PaO_2 at peak exercise due to true diffusion impairment for oxygen between the alveolar surface and erythrocytes rapidly transiting through the pulmonary circulation. The *end-tidal partial pressure of oxygen* ($P_{ET}O_2$), which serves as a surrogate measure of the alveolar

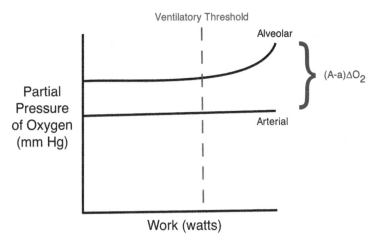

Fig. 3.2 Changes in the partial pressure of oxygen during exercise. The alveolar and arterial partial pressures of oxygen remain constant until the ventilatory threshold (*red dotted line*). After this point, the alveolar partial pressure of oxygen increases while the arterial value remains constant. As a result, the alveolar–arterial oxygen difference [$(A-a)\Delta O_2$] increases

partial pressure of oxygen (P_AO_2), changes in a different manner. This parameter remains relatively constant until the ventilatory threshold at which point it increases due to the increase in minute and alveolar ventilation (Fig. 3.1i). The rise in P_AO_2 after the ventilatory threshold would be expected to cause an increase in PaO_2, but as noted above, this is not observed. In fact, normal subjects show an increase in the *alveolar–arterial oxygen difference* [$(A-a)\Delta O_2$] with a maximum effort and, as a result, the PaO_2 remains relatively constant (Fig. 3.2).

ARTERIAL pH
The blood pH remains constant until the ventilatory threshold when it begins to fall because the increase in minute ventilation, and subsequent respiratory alkalosis, is not sufficient to fully compensate for the developing metabolic acidosis.

CARDIAC OUTPUT ($\dot{Q}$)
As work rate increases, cardiac output increases in a linear fashion before leveling off near peak exercise. As noted above, measurement of cardiac output requires invasive and time-intensive procedures, such as a pulmonary artery catheter, so direct measurements of this

parameter are not routinely obtained during a cardiopulmonary exercise test and the $\dot{V}O_{2\,max}$ is used to provide an assessment of the adequacy of cardiac output at maximum exercise.

DEAD-SPACE FRACTION (V_D/V_T)

In normal individuals at rest, V_D/V_T will initially be about 0.30–0.35. In other words, about 30–35% of minute ventilation is devoted to clearing the physiologic dead space, with the remainder available for alveolar ventilation. As individuals exercise at higher levels of power output, pulmonary blood flow increases leading to recruitment and distention of the pulmonary vasculature. This results in better matching of ventilation and perfusion and, as a result, less dead space, with V_D/V_T usually falling to between 0.10 and 0.20 by end-exercise.

HEART RATE

This increases in a linear manner as work rate or $\dot{V}O_2$ increases until peak exercise when it plateaus. On average, in normal individuals this plateau is observed near the person's age-predicted maximum heart rate (220 – age). It is important to remember that the equation used to determine the predicted maximum heart rate only represents an average response, and normal individuals may be above or below the age-predicted number by as much as 20 or 30 beats per minute (Fig. 3.1b).

The *heart rate reserve*, the difference between the maximum heart rate achieved during the test and the age-predicted maximum heart rate, is usually small (<20 bpm) in normal individuals. It is important to recognize, however, that there are large differences in maximum exercise heart rates in normal age-matched individuals. Hence although the term "reserve" is used in this context, no exercise subject has the ability to further increase his or her heart rate at maximum effort.

MINUTE VENTILATION ($\dot{V}E$)

This initially increases in a linear fashion as power output and $\dot{V}O_2$ increase. This increase is due to increases in both respiratory rate and tidal volume. With the onset of the ventilatory threshold at about two-thirds of the way through a maximum exercise effort, there is a disproportionate rise in $\dot{V}E$ compared to the power output (Fig. 3.1a), and this increase is mostly driven by an increase in respiratory rate, with tidal volume remaining steady at about 60% of the person's vital capacity (Fig. 3.1g). In normal individuals, $\dot{V}E$ at maximum exercise is usually well below the person's maximum voluntary ventilation (MVV) and we say that the person has a large "ventilatory reserve." Very fit athletes, however, will raise their minute ventilation to levels at or near their MVV.

OXYGEN SATURATION (SaO$_2$)

Given that the PaO$_2$ remains constant throughout exercise, oxygen saturation should remain constant as well. While the hemoglobin–oxygen dissociation curve does shift to the right due to the acidosis and increased temperature associated with very heavy exercise, the normal PaO$_2$ during exercise is high enough that this influence causes little to no change in the SpO$_2$ measured using a finger, forehead, or earlobe oximeter.

OXYGEN CONSUMPTION (V̇O$_2$)

This parameter increases in a linear manner as work rate increases until a plateau is reached at maximum effort (Fig. 3.1c). Individuals cannot continue to exercise for very long once they reach their V̇O$_{2\,max}$, although highly fit individuals can sustain exercise at this level longer than normal subjects. In normal individuals, V̇O$_{2\,max}$ should be ≥80% predicted for that individual based on their age, height, and gender.

PULMONARY ARTERY PRESSURE

Pulmonary artery pressure is a function of pulmonary blood flow and pulmonary vascular resistance. Despite the increase in pulmonary blood flow that occurs as cardiac output rises throughout exercise, pulmonary artery pressure rises to only a modest extent because increased pulmonary blood flow leads to recruitment and distention of the pulmonary vasculature, which, in turn, decreases pulmonary vascular resistance. Because measurement of this parameter requires a pulmonary artery catheter, measurement is not done as part of an ordinary exercise test and, instead, is performed only in very specific circumstances.

RESPIRATORY EXCHANGE RATIO (R)

R is the ratio of carbon dioxide output to oxygen consumption (V̇CO$_2$ / V̇O$_2$). At rest this value depends on the balance between fat and carbohydrate metabolism, and usually ranges from 0.8 to 0.9. With increasing levels of exercise, carbohydrate utilization becomes a progressively larger fraction of the metabolic fuel. As a result, R increases progressively. After the onset of the ventilatory threshold, V̇CO$_2$ rises to a greater extent than V̇O$_2$ and R rapidly rises to levels as high as 1.1–1.3 (Fig. 3.1h). This additional increase in V̇CO$_2$ takes place as the compensatory hyperventilation of maximum exercise starts to wash out body CO$_2$ stores. Following cessation of exercise, R continues to rise because V̇O$_2$ declines significantly, while the individual continues to eliminate significant amounts of CO_2 that was produced and transiently stored in the exercising muscle.

STROKE VOLUME

During upright exercise, two pumps facilitate cardiac output: the heart pumping blood into the aorta, and the calf capacitance veins and their valves, pumping blood from the legs back into the vena cava. Stroke volume, which as noted above is estimated using the O_2 pulse, increases with the onset of exercise, primarily because of the mobilization of blood in the venous capacitance vessels in the legs while in the later stages of exercise stroke volume increases only minimally as a result of increased inotropic activity (Fig. 3.1b).

SYSTEMIC BLOOD PRESSURE

This parameter increases with exercise due to a rise in cardiac output and increase in vascular resistance in the renal, splanchnic, and skin circulations. In normal individuals, there is usually a step-change in the systolic pressure near the ventilatory threshold, after which systemic pressure can often reach very high levels. In fact, it is not uncommon for normal individuals to have systolic pressures rise into the 200 mmHg range at peak exercise. Diastolic pressure will ordinarily decrease modestly throughout exercise, reflecting vasodilation of the exercising muscle beds.

TIDAL VOLUME (VT)

The tidal volume (VT) increases until around the time of the ventilatory threshold after which time it tends to level off at about 60% of the individual's vital capacity (Fig. 3.1g).

VENTILATORY EQUIVALENT FOR CARBON DIOXIDE ($\dot{V}E/\dot{V}CO_2$)

This ratio, which reflects the amount of ventilation expended per liter of CO_2 exhaled, is typically between 24 and 34 at rest and remains in that range until after the ventilatory threshold, after which it increases (Fig. 3.1f). This is because minute ventilation is rising at a faster rate than CO_2 production. Occasionally, highly fit athletes or anxious individuals will hyperventilate during rest or unloaded pedaling, which raises these values above the expected range. Once exercise starts, however, the ventilatory equivalent for these individuals will typically decline back to the expected range and follow the typical pattern for the normal individual.

VENTILATORY EQUIVALENT FOR OXYGEN ($\dot{V}E/\dot{V}CO_2$)

This ratio, which represents the amount of ventilation necessary to take in a given amount of oxygen, follows a very similar trend as the $\dot{V}E/\dot{V}CO_2$, although the point where it increases is the true ventilatory threshold (Fig. 3.1f). Values are typically 22–32 at rest and remain in that range until the ventilatory threshold, at which point they rise to higher levels because minute ventilation is now rising at a faster rate than oxygen consumption. As with $\dot{V}E/\dot{V}CO_2$, higher than expected values can also be seen at rest and during unloaded pedaling in highly fit athletes or anxious individuals. These values will return to the normal range once the individual begins exercise against resistance.

THE EFFECTS OF TRAINING AND GENETICS IN NORMAL INDIVIDUALS

Normal individuals can increase the distance they can walk, climb, or ride in a given time period as a result of a training regimen. However, while the increases in muscle strength and endurance with training programs can be significant, the improvement achieved in $\dot{V}O_{2\,max}$ is relatively modest. Generally, an unfit subject can increase his or her $\dot{V}O_{2\,max}$ by about 15% with intensive training over several months. However, regardless of the duration or rigor of the training effort, you cannot take a "couch potato" with an average $\dot{V}O_{2\,max}$ and create an Olympic-level cross-country skier with a very high $\dot{V}O_{2\,max}$. Likewise even fit athletes with a very high $\dot{V}O_{2\,max}$ at baseline cannot do much to increase their $\dot{V}O_{2\,max}$ with more intensive training. What improves with intensive training is exercise efficiency, the ability to sustain high work rates for prolonged periods of time, and the ability to recover quickly from repeated sets of maximum exercise.

The fact that you cannot "train-up" someone's $\dot{V}O_{2\,max}$ from an average to an elite level implies that a good part of someone's exercise capacity is heritable and reflects what one's parents could do. Interestingly, there also appears to be a "heritability of trainability" in which how much one can improve with training is also a reflection of how much one's parents could achieve in a training regimen.

EXERCISE RESPONSES IN PATIENTS WITH DECREASED EXERCISE CAPACITY

One of the cardinal manifestations of various diseases is dyspnea on exertion. Although many patients discount the importance of this symptom and do not perceive loss of exercise tolerance as a significant problem, diminished exercise tolerance is one of the most sensitive markers of cardiopulmonary disease, and questions about exercise tolerance should be part of any screening medical history.

As noted earlier, decreased exercise tolerance can occur as a result of problems in one of several systems including the respiratory system, the cardiovascular system, and the neuromuscular system. In some cases, multiple systems are concurrently responsible for the decreased exercise tolerance but one of the systems can usually be identified as having the predominant role. When patients have decreased exercise capacity due to problems in one of these systems, the physiologic responses to exercise tend to deviate from the patterns described above for normal individuals. Importantly, depending on the particular system that is primarily responsible for the decrease in exercise tolerance, the physiologic parameters deviate in characteristic patterns that can be differentiated from each other.

We will describe the characteristic patterns of physiologic responses that are seen when patients have limited exercise capacity, focusing on the ventilatory pump, gas exchange in the lungs, the heart, and the pulmonary vascular system. The key findings in each pattern of limitation are summarized in Table 3.1 and are described in greater detail below. As you read these descriptions of the characteristic physiologic responses, you should be aware that these represent idealized versions of these patterns. In actual clinical practice, patients may demonstrate all or just some of these features during a progressive work exercise test. As will be discussed later in Chap. 5, the variability in presentations needs to be taken into account when determining the cause of a patient's exercise limitation. Rather than making decisions based on the presence or the absence of a single variable, you need to look at the constellation of variables to see if they fit one of the patterns below.

TABLE 3.1 KEY FINDINGS FOR THE BASIC PATTERNS OF EXERCISE LIMITATION

| Variable | Patterns of limitation | | |
	Cardiac[a]	Pulmonary vascular disease/ILD[b]	Ventilatory
Blood pressure	Should rise throughout[c]	Rises throughout	Rises throughout
Dead space (V_D/V_T)[d]	Decreases	Remains stable or increases	Variable decrease[e]
Heart rate reserve	Variable	Small to absent	Large
Metabolic acidosis (late exercise)	Present	Present	Absent
O_2 pulse	May plateau near end-exercise	May plateau near end-exercise	Increases throughout[f]
Oxygen saturation	Stable	May decrease	May decrease
$P_{ET}CO_2$ (late exercise)	Decreased	Decreased	Increased or stable
Reason for stopping	Leg fatigue	Dyspnea, leg fatigue	Dyspnea
Respiratory exchange ratio	Usually exceeds 1.1	Usually exceeds 1.1	Often remains below 1.0
$\dot{V}E / \dot{V}CO_2$	May be increased[g]	Increased[h]	Increased[i]
Ventilatory reserve	Large	Small	Small–Absent
Ventilatory threshold	Present	Present	Absent
$\dot{V}O_{2max}$	Decreased[j]	Decreased	Decreased

Variables have been listed in alphabetical order rather than according to importance in determining the cause of exercise limitation

[a]The normal individual will demonstrate a "cardiac pattern" of limitation. The key factor that distinguishes them from someone with underlying cardiac disease is the fact that the $\dot{V}O_{2max}$ will be in the normal range whereas it will be decreased in an individual with underlying cardiac disease

[b]Interstitial lung disease patients demonstrate a pattern very similar to the pulmonary vascular pattern and can only be differentiated based on their Pulmonary function tests (PFTs) and chest imaging

[c]In some patients with underlying cardiac disease, blood pressure may not rise or may even decrease with progressive exercise, a concerning finding indicative of severe disease

[d]As measured by arterial blood gases. This yields a different and more diagnostically useful value than that reported by many exercise systems that use the end-tidal CO_2 instead of arterial CO_2 in the calculation

[e]V_D/V_T may not decrease in patients who develop severe air-trapping during exercise

[f]Patients with ventilatory limitation may have a plateau in their O_2 pulse if they have severe air-trapping

[g]Increased ventilatory equivalents noted before the ventilatory threshold are suggestive of severe heart failure

[h]This is suggestive of increased dead-space

[i]Seen with severe chronic obstructive pulmonary disease with carbon dioxide retention

[j]Normal individuals also demonstrate a cardiac pattern of limitation. The $\dot{V}O_{2max}$ in these individuals will be in the normal range as predicted by their age, gender, and height

CARDIAC LIMITATION

In patients with valvular or ischemic cardiomyopathy, the heart is the limiting factor in exercise. Exercise capacity is diminished because the heart cannot deliver enough oxygen-rich blood to the exercising muscles. The $\dot{V}O_{2\,max}$ will be reduced relative to age-, gender-, and height-matched normal individuals. At any given work rate or $\dot{V}O_2$, the heart rate may be increased relative to normals, indicating that the stroke volume is likely decreased. At peak exercise, the heart rate may reach their age-predicted maximum, but most cardiac diseases also cause a chronotropic limitation, in which case their heart rate at maximum exercise is well below their age-predicted maximum. The O_2 pulse typically reaches a plateau in late exercise at a level below that which you would predict for the individual.

With any maximum cardiac effort, a ventilatory threshold is always observed at about two-thirds of the way through the exercise performance, regardless of the maximum heart rate achieved. Although minute ventilation ($\dot{V}E$) is typically higher at any given work rate for the most impaired individuals compared to normal subjects, there is still a large reserve between $\dot{V}E$ at peak exercise and the patient's MVV. Therefore, patients with severe cardiomyopathy often demonstrate higher ventilatory equivalents for oxygen and carbon dioxide. Oxygen saturation typically remains normal during exercise and the dead-space fraction decreases as it does with normal subjects. In some patients with severe ischemic heart disease, blood pressure will not increase as expected with exercise. In severe cardiomyopathy, blood pressure may even fall and is an indication to abort an exercise test. ST segment changes may also be observed on electrocardiography and, when present, are highly suggestive of cardiac limitation. Patients with a primary cardiac limitation, like normal subjects, usually stop exercising because of symptoms of leg fatigue.

This pattern of results is often referred to as a "cardiac limitation" pattern and is demonstrated graphically in the form of a 9-Box plot in Fig. 3.3. The pattern for the individual with cardiac disease is displayed in this figure along with the responses in a normal individual in order to make it easier to appreciate the characteristic findings.

It is important to remember that all normal individuals also display a cardiac pattern. This is because these "normals" are also limited by the amount of oxygenated blood that can be delivered to exercising muscle by their heart. Both normal individuals and those with heart disease will reach their ventilatory threshold at about two-thirds of their maximum effort. What distinguishes the exercise test pattern of a normal person from a person with cardiac disease with the same age, gender, and height is that the normal person will achieve

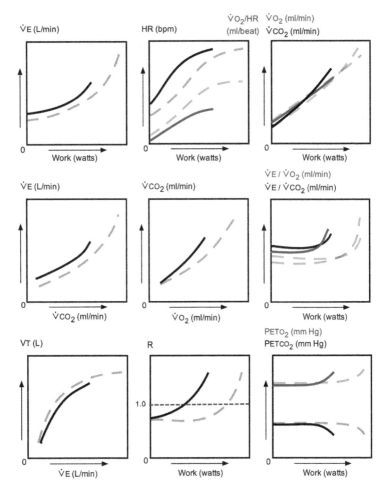

Fig. 3.3 9-Box plot demonstrating characteristic changes seen in patients with cardiac limitation due to underlying cardiac disease (*solid lines*) compared to normal individuals (*dotted lines*)

a higher work rate and $\dot{V}O_{2\,max}$. There are also differences in the absolute values of certain variables such as the ventilatory equivalents for oxygen and carbon dioxide, heart rate, and O_2 pulse, but the general pattern of change in these variables will be similar between normal individuals and those with cardiac disease.

VENTILATORY LIMITATION

Patients with chronic obstructive pulmonary disease (COPD) or severe asthma have altered ventilatory mechanics that limit their exercise capacity well before they reach the limits of their cardiac performance. In other words, the ventilatory pump fails well before the heart does. At any given work rate, $\dot{V}E$ is higher than in normals, as the result of increased dead-space ventilation. At peak exercise, $\dot{V}E$ is at or just below their MVV indicating that they have no ventilatory reserve. In an individual with ventilatory limitation due to severe obstructive lung disease, the tidal volume may actually decrease in late exercise as the individual develops progressive air-trapping.

Instead of the expected decrease in $PaCO_2$ with maximum exercise, patients with ventilatory limitation develop a respiratory acidosis because they cannot generate enough alveolar ventilation to eliminate the CO_2 being produced in exercising muscles. Heart rate rises with exercise but because ventilatory failure occurs before the heart is stressed to its maximum, peak heart rate will ordinarily be well below the age-predicted maximum (i.e., a large "heart rate reserve"). Be aware that not every case of large heart rate reserve can be attributed to ventilatory limitation. Some patients have cardiac limitation due to chronotropic incompetence alone and hence will demonstrate a large "heart rate reserve" (although in that instance, the heart is incapable of generating a faster rate).

Because ventilatory mechanics limit the person before their heart reaches its limit, the heart is able to meet the blood flow demands of the exercising muscle. As a result, significant lactic acidosis does not develop and you cannot identify a ventilatory threshold. The absence of the ventilatory threshold and a rising $PaCO_2$ are hallmarks of ventilatory exercise limitation. Oxygen saturation may fall due to areas of lung with low ventilation–perfusion ratios.

The $\dot{V}O_{2\,max}$ will be reduced relative to age-, gender-, and height-matched normal individuals. Although a plateau in the O_2 pulse is commonly associated with cardiac limitation, this finding can also be seen in patients with ventilatory limitation due to severe obstructive lung disease. In these cases, the patients develop severe air-trapping due to inadequate exhalation time which, in turn, leads to increased intrathoracic pressure, decreased venous return, and decreased stroke volume. These patients stop exercising with a primary complaint of dyspnea.

The ventilatory pattern of limitation is described graphically in Fig. 3.4.

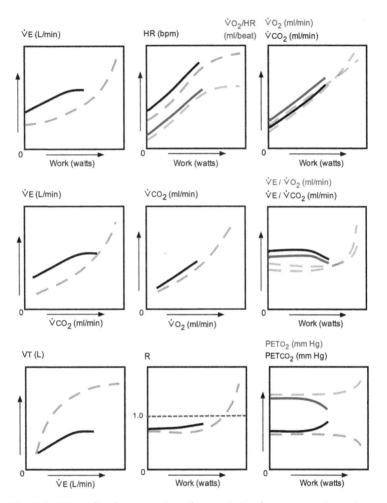

Fig. 3.4 9-Box plot demonstrating characteristic changes seen in patients with ventilatory limitation (*solid lines*) compared to normal individuals who demonstrate a cardiac pattern of limitation (*dotted lines*)

LIMITATION DUE TO PULMONARY VASCULAR DISEASE OR INTERSTITIAL LUNG DISEASE

Although pulmonary vascular diseases, such as idiopathic pulmonary arterial hypertension, and interstitial lung diseases (ILD), such as idiopathic pulmonary fibrosis, are different pathophysiologic entities, patients with these underlying diseases tend to demonstrate similar

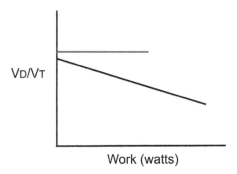

Fig. 3.5 Changes in the dead-space fraction in individuals with a pulmonary vascular/interstitial lung disease pattern of limitation (*red line*) compared to normal individuals (*black line*). Note that the patient with the pulmonary vascular/interstitial lung disease pattern of limitation stops exercising at a lower level of power output than the normal individual

patterns of physiologic responses during progressive exercise. For this reason, we tend to consider them as a single category of exercise limitation which we call the pulmonary vascular/interstitial lung disease pattern.

In many respects, the pattern of physiologic responses looks similar to that of the patient with cardiac limitation. Heart rate rises as expected with increasing exercise intensity but is typically much higher at any given level of work than in normals. The $\dot{V}O_{2\,max}$ is reduced relative to age-, gender-, and height-matched normal individuals and a ventilatory threshold can be identified because right heart dysfunction in the face of the pulmonary vascular disease impairs cardiac output to the point that the heart cannot meet the blood flow demands of exercising muscle and lactic acidosis develops. What sets the pulmonary vascular/ILD pattern apart from cardiac limitation are two key physiologic responses. First, due to changes in the pulmonary vasculature, these patients cannot recruit previously unused pulmonary vessels as cardiac output rises. As a result, the dead-space fraction remains at or near resting levels as exercise intensity increases and pulmonary artery pressure increases significantly (Fig. 3.5). Second, the diseased lung is less able to oxygenate returning blood that has a low mixed venous oxygen content, and the increasing blood flow relative to ventilation creates more regions with low ventilation–perfusion ratios and a subsequent fall in PaO_2 and SaO_2, values which normally remain constant in the cardiac limitation pattern.

Because pulmonary vascular and interstitial lung disease patients can look very similar on cardiopulmonary exercise testing, additional studies such as echocardiography, pulmonary function testing, and chest imaging are necessary to distinguish the different disease entities.

The pulmonary vascular/interstitial lung disease pattern of limitation is described graphically in Fig. 3.6.

MISCELLANEOUS PATTERNS OF EXERCISE LIMITATION

The majority of patients in whom you perform cardiopulmonary exercise tests will demonstrate physiologic responses consistent with one of the three patterns described above. In some cases, however, it will be difficult to label a patient as having one of these primary patterns and you will need to consider alternative explanations for the observed exercise responses. Among the wide variety of problems that fall within this category, two particular problems that warrant mention include the following:

Poor Effort

Some patients will not give a full effort during the cardiopulmonary exercise test. This might occur because they are malingering or because they stop early secondary to severe pain in their hips or knees. When patients do not give a full effort, in addition to the fact that $\dot{V}O_{2\,max}$ is reduced relative to age-, gender-, and height-matched normal individuals there is no identifiable ventilatory threshold and the respiratory exchange ratio does not rise above 1.0, even in the post exercise state. The patient's maximum heart rate and maximum ventilation will also typically be well below the predicted values for the individual.

Neuromuscular Diseases

While the neuromuscular system is an important link in the overall physiologic response to exercise, patients with the diverse abnormalities included under this category usually are not sent for CPET testing because diagnostic abnormalities have already been identified in the process of a neurological workup. Hence this is an unusual indication for exercise testing. In patients in whom neuromuscular disease is the predominant factor limiting exercise tolerance, the muscles fail before either the ventilatory pump or the heart reach the limits of their capacity. As a result, in addition to the fact that $\dot{V}O_{2\,max}$ is reduced relative to age-, gender-, and height-matched normal individuals, the patient will have both increased heart rate and ventilatory reserves; heart rate and minute ventilation both rise with increasing exercise

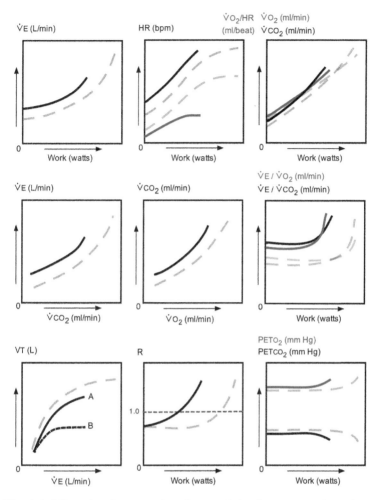

Fig. 3.6 9-Box plot demonstrating characteristic changes seen in patients with a pulmonary vascular/interstitial lung disease pattern of limitation (*solid lines*) compared to normal individuals who demonstrate a cardiac pattern of limitation (*dotted lines*). In the graph in the *lower left-hand corner* (VT vs. V̇E), the *solid black line* (A) represents the expected response for a patient with pulmonary vascular disease while the *dotted black line* (B) represents the expected response for a patient with interstitial lung disease

intensity but at peak exercise will be well below the age-predicted maximum heart rate and MVV, respectively. In most cases, a ventilatory threshold is not observed because the neuromuscular system is failing well before the heart has reached the limits of its ability to deliver blood to the muscles. The respiratory exchange ratio (R) often fails to increase above 1.0 for similar reasons.

In many respects, with the large heart rate and ventilatory reserves, R that remains near or below 1.0 and the absent ventilatory threshold, this pattern looks a lot like the patient who does not give a full effort on their exercise test. The distinction between poor effort and the neuromuscular pattern will largely be made based on observing the patient carefully through the test, looking for evidence of dyspnea, sweating, and other factors that suggest they gave a strong effort. This is described in greater detail in Chap. 4.

The reader should keep in mind that there are a wide variety of neuromuscular diseases with different clinical manifestations. As a result, there can be a wide variety of exercise responses and patients with such diseases may not fit the pattern described here. For example, some patients with prominent respiratory muscle involvement may demonstrate a rising $P_{ET}CO_2$ in late exercise and have a pattern more consistent with ventilatory limitation. Because of this variability it is difficult to identify one specific exercise pattern consistent with all neuromuscular diseases.

Patients with other disease processes such as severe peripheral vascular disease with claudication, metabolic disorders, and mitochondrial myopathies may also demonstrate patterns of exercise responses that do not fit neatly within the three major patterns of exercise limitation described earlier. Because these problems are uncommon and because the underlying disease will often be identified through other diagnostic testing, we will not emphasize these miscellaneous processes further and will focus the remainder of the text on identifying the most common causes of exercise limitation.

THE EFFECT OF TRAINING IN PATIENTS WITH UNDERLYING DISEASE

When people have exercise limitation for one of the broad reasons described above, training programs may yield benefits for them including improvements in their maximum exercise capacity as well as in their ability to sustain and tolerate physical work. For example, pulmonary rehabilitation programs have been extensively studied in patients with COPD and have been demonstrated to improve multiple outcomes including exercise capacity, perceived intensity of breathlessness, and quality of life while decreasing hospitalizations and depression. Hence although these programs have not been demonstrated to improve mortality, they are safe and do improve overall functional capacity, even though ventilatory capacity or cardiac output may remain unchanged.

REFERENCE

1. Wasserman K, Hansen JE, Sue DY, Stringer WW, Whipp BJ. Principles of exercise testing and interpretation. 4th ed. Philadelphia, PA: Lippincott, Williams and Wilkins; 2005.

Chapter 4
Conducting a Cardiopulmonary Exercise Test

Keywords Angina • Aortic stenosis • Arterial blood gases • Arterial catheter • Asthma • Arrhythmia • Beta-blockers • Contraindications • Coronary artery disease • Cycle ergometer • Defibrillator • Dyspnea • Electrocardiogram • Hypertrophic obstructive cardiomyopathy • Hypoxemia • Indications • Myocardial ischemia • Myocardial infarction • Pacemaker • Pregnancy • Pulmonary edema • Pulmonary embolism • Ramp • Syncope • Treadmill • Work rate

CONDUCTING A CARDIOPULMONARY EXERCISE TEST

In many institutions, the person responsible for interpreting the cardiopulmonary exercise test will also be the person supervising the test as it takes place. As part of this role, there are tasks that must be addressed before, during, and after the test is completed.

The responsibilities described below represent the practice at our institution. Because some of these specific tasks may vary from institution to institution, if a trainee is conducting the test, he or she should meet with their supervising practitioner in advance of their first studies to clarify the usual procedures performed in a test.

A.M. Luks et al., *Introduction to Cardiopulmonary Exercise Testing*, DOI 10.1007/978-1-4614-6283-5_4, © Springer Science+Business Media New York 2013

BEFORE THE TEST

REVIEW THE INDICATIONS FOR THE TEST

It is important to review the request form for the study as well as the requesting provider's clinic notes to be sure that you understand the purpose of the test as, this may affect decisions about which data to collect or other aspects of the study. For example, when a patient is referred for evaluation of dyspnea on exertion of unclear etiology, it may be useful to obtain arterial blood gases during the test to help rule in or out the possibility of pulmonary vascular disease (the reasoning for this is discussed further below). On the other hand, a patient sent from the heart failure clinic for serial evaluation of their $\dot{V}O_{2\,max}$ does not require blood gases in most cases because the etiology of their exercise limitation is already known and the requesting provider is simply trying to follow the progression of their disease. In general, the primary reasons why exercise tests are performed include the following:

- *Identify the etiology of dyspnea on exertion or exercise limitation*: There are two situations in which this applies: (1) a patient has experienced a progressive loss of exercise capacity but has multiple potential etiologies (e.g., are they limited by their chronic obstructive pulmonary disease (COPD) or by their coronary artery disease); (2) a patient has progressive exertional limitation that remains unexplained after clinical evaluation, laboratory tests, radiography, and pulmonary function testing.
- *Follow progression of disease*: Physicians caring for patients with advanced cardiomyopathies often follow their patient's $\dot{V}O_{2\,max}$ in a serial manner to guide decisions about when to list the patient for transplant. An adult congenital heart disease provider might use the test for similar purposes or to decide when other surgical procedures are necessary.
- *Monitoring the effects of therapy*
- *To determine fitness for surgical procedures such as lung resection*
- *Participation in research protocols*

REVIEW WHETHER ANY CONTRAINDICATIONS EXIST

To avoid adverse patient events during the test, it is critical to review whether the patient has any contraindications to undergoing testing.

Absolute contraindications to cardiopulmonary exercise testing include: [1]

- Active myocardial ischemia (unstable angina, myocardial infarction within 30 days)
- Acute heart failure exacerbation
- Exercise-induced syncope
- Uncontrolled arrhythmias
- Severe aortic stenosis
- Acute endocarditis, myocarditis, pericarditis
- Acute aortic dissection
- Acute pulmonary embolism or lower extremity venous thromboembolism
- Active COPD exacerbation or uncontrolled asthma
- Pulmonary edema
- Suspected dissecting aortic aneurysm

Relative contraindications include: [1]

- Severe pulmonary hypertension
- Left main coronary artery stenosis
- Moderate stenotic valvular disease
- Severe hypertension (SBP > 200 mmHg, DBP > 120 mmHg)
- Hypertrophic cardiomyopathy
- High-degree atrioventricular block
- Severe electrolyte abnormalities
- Tachy- or brady-arrhythmias
- Advanced or complicated pregnancy
- Implanted cardiac defibrillator that cannot be interrogated or temporarily reset due to inaccessibility of an individual qualified to do this (e.g., device manufacturer representative).

If there is any uncertainty as to the patient's suitability for cardiopulmonary exercise testing, trainees should contact a supervising attending physician prior to initiating the testing protocol.

OBTAIN OTHER IMPORTANT CLINICAL INFORMATION FROM THE PATIENT

Before the test you should also review whether the patient is on any relevant cardiac or pulmonary medications or has undergone any cardiac or thoracic surgical procedures. This information will be noted in your final report.

OBTAIN CONSENT FOR THE TEST FROM THE PATIENT

As with all procedures performed on patients, it is necessary to explain the risks and benefits of the procedure to the patient and obtain informed consent. The main risks you need to impart to the patient include breathlessness, leg fatigue, myocardial ischemia, hypoxemia, syncope, arrhythmia, and death. The risk of death from a cardiopulmonary exercise test is 1:10,000 for a population being evaluated for possible coronary artery disease. The risk is likely increased in patients with diseases listed above under the relative contraindications list. The primary benefits will depend on why the physician ordered the test.

It is important to tell the patient that useful data will not be obtained from the test unless they give a full effort. As a result, they should expect to get very tired and should try to push through that sensation until they cannot go anymore. They should be encouraged to do their best and stop only when they feel they must do so. The patient should be reassured that their dyspnea will resolve once the test is completed and that the laboratory has the resources to deal with any of the complications noted above.

CHECK FOR NECESSARY PERSONNEL AND EQUIPMENT
Advanced cardiac life support (ACLS) competent personnel and a cart containing all necessary ACLS equipment, including a defibrillator, must be readily available in the testing laboratory.

RESET THRESHOLDS ON IMPLANTED DEFIBRILLATORS
Some patients referred for cardiopulmonary exercise testing will have implanted defibrillators. In such cases, it is important that the device does not deliver inappropriate shocks in response to elevated heart rates that occur during the exercise period, but still delivers appropriate shocks if the patient has an arrhythmia such as ventricular tachycardia or ventricular fibrillation. The person conducting the test should contact the cardiologist or electrophysiologist caring for the patient to confirm that the defibrillator settings can be temporarily changed, as well as recommended settings if a change is permissible. A representative from the defibrillator manufacturer can then implement the recommended change, being careful to allow the defibrillator to still shock in appropriate situations. This person should be notified well ahead of the test to avoid unnecessary delays on the day of testing. At the conclusion of the test, the defibrillator should be reset to its original settings.

DETERMINE IF SUPPLEMENTAL OXYGEN IS NEEDED
Patients on home oxygen and other patients with severe COPD will usually exercise with supplemental oxygen to prevent profound hypoxemia. Patients cannot wear their nasal cannula during the exercise test and special equipment is needed to provide supplemental

oxygen during the test. If you are unsure about whether to use supplemental oxygen, you should consult with the supervising physician and the laboratory technicians. You should also be aware that most exercise systems have difficulty accurately measuring oxygen consumption when the subject is on fraction of inspired oxygen higher than air. The accuracy problem arises because of small leaks of ambient air into the inspired oxygen mix, giving an inappropriately high measurement of oxygen consumption.

PLACE AN ARTERIAL CATHETER IF INDICATED

Arterial blood gases are not required for every study, but are useful in situations where pulmonary vascular disease or interstitial lung disease is a diagnostic possibility. As was discussed in Chap. 3, one of the defining features of the pulmonary vascular/interstitial lung disease pattern of limitation in cardiopulmonary exercise testing is that the dead-space fraction (V_D/V_T) fails to decrease with progressive exercise. Calculation of the dead-space fraction requires arterial blood gases. Some cardiopulmonary exercise testing systems provide a calculated V_D/V_T based on exhaled gas values, but arterial blood gases are required for accurate determination of this parameter. Exercise blood gases also allow you to definitively state whether the subject developed a metabolic acidosis, had a ventilatory limitation, and achieved a ventilatory threshold (discussed further in Chap. 5).

While it is possible to obtain blood gases by arterial punctures at the start and end of a test, placement of an indwelling arterial catheter allows you to obtain serial measurements and obviates the need to do individual radial artery sticks, which can be quite challenging in an exercising patient who cannot keep their arm still. This is particularly important with regard to the blood gas done at the conclusion of the test, as this must be obtained within 1 minute of completing exercise in order for the data to be useful. You should also be aware that following exercise, patients are more likely to have a vagal response to needlesticks and could develop syncope during the attempt to obtain the blood gas in this manner.

DETERMINE THE "RAMP"

When we perform cardiopulmonary exercise tests to determine the etiology of dyspnea on exertion, we use a protocol referred to as an "incremental test to a symptom-limited maximum." Another term for this, as noted earlier in this text, is the progressive work exercise test. This type of test is distinct from a constant work rate test in which the test subject cycles on an ergometer or walks/runs on a treadmill at a constant work rate for the duration of the test.

When performing an incremental test to symptom-limited maximum, it is necessary to determine the rate at which the work rate will increase during the test, a variable referred to as "the ramp." The work rate can rise in continuous fashion (i.e., linear increase in work rate over time) or can be increased in stepwise increments each minute. At our institution, we prefer to use a continuously increasing work rate.

The goal in choosing the ramp is to pick a rate of rise in the work rate that will require about 10 minutes of exercise for the subject to reach their symptom-limited maximum effort. If they are placed on too steep a ramp (i.e., the work rate increases too quickly), it is difficult to identify a ventilatory threshold and your maximum measured $\dot{V}O_2$ may be less than the true $\dot{V}O_{2max}$. Choosing too slow a ramp (i.e., the work rate increases too slowly) is not as problematic but does risk tiring the patient out before they reach what should be their maximum exercise capacity. Obese patients may also overheat and not be able to manifest their true $\dot{V}O_{2max}$. It is not necessary for the test subject to cycle for exactly 10 minutes but it is helpful for them to exercise for close to this time.

ESTIMATING THE RAMP FOR TESTS USING CYCLE ERGOMETRY

If the cardiopulmonary exercise test is being conducted using a cycle ergometer, the ramp can be anywhere from 5 to 30 W/minute, with the number varying in increments of 5 W/minute (e.g., 5, 10, 15, ...). While there are formal ways to determine the ramp based on prediction equations that take into account physical characteristics of the patient, such as age, height, weight, and gender [2], we prefer to use a less formal approach that we have found to work well in the majority of patients. This method involves asking the patient about their activities at home and using their answers as a guide to pick the ramp. To employ this method, you can take advantage of the fact that in the majority of individuals, the ability to carry out certain types of physical activity corresponds to certain maximum oxygen consumption values. These questions, therefore, allow you to estimate the $\dot{V}O_{2max}$ of the patient which can then be used to determine the ramp. Table 4.1 lists the approximate $\dot{V}O_{2max}$ values associated with particular levels of exercise tolerance and the appropriate ramps for these patients.

When using these guidelines, it is important to adjust your chosen ramp based on the person's body size. For very small subjects, you

TABLE 4.1 ESTIMATING THE PATIENT'S $\dot{V}O_{2MAX}$ BASED ON THE PATIENT'S ACTIVITY TOLERANCE

Approximate activity level	Estimated $\dot{V}O_{2max}$ (ml/kg/minute)	Approximate ramp (W/minute)
Able to participate in competitive sports with sustained activity like rowing, basketball, and soccer. Engages in regular, endurance training	>40	25–30
Tolerates sustained heavy labor well; can play recreational soccer or full-court basketball without slacking or run at an 8 minute/mile place	35–40	20
Recreational cross-country skiing or half-court basketball with minimal limitation	30–35	20
Heavy labor with difficulty; downhill skiing somewhat limited by fatigue	25–30	15
Heavy housework or yard work causes dyspnea; cannot play singles tennis	20–25	15
Dyspnea with two flights of stairs at own pace; cannot play golf while carrying bag or pulling a cart	17–20	10
Unable to vacuum average room or change sheets without rest	14–17	10
Difficulty walking slowly with peers in shopping mall	12–14	5
Dyspnea while brushing hair, dressing, showering	<12	5

should subtract 5 W/minute. For obese patients, you should add 5 W/minute to your ramp and for very obese people you should add 10 W/minute to the ramp. These adjustments are made with obese patients because the cardiac output and oxygen consumption an obese person requires to even walk slowly on the level may be two to three times that required by a person with normal body weight. This difference is even more dramatic with any activity that requires walking uphill or upstairs.

In well-muscled, highly fit individuals, it is appropriate to use a 30 W/minute increment but do not be surprised if they continue exercising well beyond 10 minute. In patients who have previously performed exercise tests in your laboratory, you can use the ramp from their prior study as a guide for picking the ramp in the current study.

This less structured approach is easier to implement in the laboratory than the formalized approaches employing prediction equations. Even though the former may not be as precise as the latter, over- or underestimation of the ramp for a patient by a small amount will not affect the measured $\dot{V}O_{2max}$, only the time the subject exercises on the cycle ergometer.

ESTIMATING THE RAMP FOR TESTS USING A TREADMILL

Incremental tests to symptom-limited maximum can also be performed on a treadmill. One of the challenges with the treadmill, however, is that it is harder to quantify the work rate than it is on a bicycle. In addition, it can also be harder to achieve a linear increase in work rate, as is done with cycle ergometry because, given the way most treadmill systems work, increases in the grade of the treadmill—one of the basic means by increasing the work rate—are difficult to achieve in a continuous manner.

Different protocols have been described for increasing the work rate during treadmill-based cardiopulmonary exercise tests. In some protocols, treadmill speed is kept constant while the grade increases by a constant amount each minute. Subjects may walk anywhere from 0.5 to 4.5 mph, depending on their assessed level of physical fitness, while the grade increases by 1–3% each minute until the subject reaches exhaustion [2, 3]. A commonly used protocol that follows this approach is the Balke protocol in which treadmill speed is kept constant at 3.3 mph while treadmill grade is increased 1% per minute [4]. Other protocols involve changing both the speed and grade of the treadmill. A commonly used example of this approach is the Bruce protocol [5] which begins with 3-minute stages of walking at 1.7 mph at grades of 0%, 5%, and 10%, followed by 3-minute stages in which the grade is increased by 2% and the speed increased by 0.8 mph. When the treadmill reaches 18% grade and 5 mph, the grade is kept constant and the speed increases by 0.5 mph. More recently, Porszasz et al. [6] described an approach that uses linear increases in speed coupled with linear increases in grade in order to achieve a linear increase in work rate.

For all treadmill protocols, recall that obese patients will have a disproportionately high oxygen consumption at any treadmill grade and speed relative to normal individuals, and generally will require the use of minimal increases in grade and speed to complete 10 minute of exercise.

DURING THE TEST

The general structure of the test is as follows: Subjects initially sit at rest on the bicycle hooked up to the monitoring equipment with the mouthpiece or the mask in place for a set period of time. We collect 3 minute of data with the patient at rest, but the particular time may vary between laboratories. Patients should not talk during this period. They will then complete another set period of unloaded pedaling (2 minute in our laboratory) before application of resistance begins. The test subject should pedal at 60–70 rpm throughout the unloaded and loaded pedaling periods and continue pedaling until they cannot pedal any longer (described further below). Some subjects—particularly very fit athletes—will prefer to cycle at higher rpm values. This deviation from the usual protocol is acceptable provided the pedal speed is kept relatively constant throughout the test.

OBTAIN BLOOD PRESSURE MEASUREMENTS

You should obtain blood pressure measurements regularly (every 2 minute in our protocol). Measurements with manual cuffs may be very difficult when the patient is exercising, as there is a lot of extra noise that interferes with your ability to detect the Korotkoff sounds. Sometimes you cannot hear the sounds and must solely rely on your ability to feel the arterial pulse as the cuff inflates and deflates. Having the subject rest their hand on your shoulder during the measurements can sometimes be helpful. This is very important data, as a fall in systolic blood pressure with increasing work rate is an indication to stop the test and is, in fact, a reliable sign of life-threatening coronary artery disease.

OBTAIN ARTERIAL BLOOD GASES

If you place an arterial line, blood gases are drawn from the catheter at preset intervals. In our laboratory, we draw these samples every 2 minute. The process of preparing the syringes, drawing blood, and flushing the catheter is fairly time consuming; so if you are doing this, you will need someone else to measure blood pressure for you unless you have an automated blood pressure monitoring system.

OBSERVE THE ELECTROCARDIOGRAM

Patients are attached to continuous 12-lead electrocardiogram (ECG) monitoring systems throughout the cardiopulmonary exercise test. An important task during the test is to observe this tracing for evidence of ischemia or concerning arrhythmias, which might warrant stopping the test before the test subject reaches maximum exercise. Intermittent premature beats (either atrial or ventricular in origin) can be tolerated but short bursts of ventricular tachycardia, sustained ventricular tachycardia, supraventricular tachycardia, or marked ST depression (≥2 mm) are indications to stop the test. Bigeminy is commonly seen in early exercise but can resolve with increasing work and is not a reason to stop a test. Be aware that significant arrhythmias frequently manifest in the immediate cool down period after exercise is completed. This is one of the main reasons a patient should not be left unobserved immediately after the test.

OBSERVING THE PATIENT
While it is very easy to focus all of your attention on the data output from the various monitors attached to the patient during the test, it is important to observe the patient too, as there are important clues to whether they gave a maximum effort and may be signs that a test should be terminated.

You should periodically ask if they are having chest pain, leg pain, lightheadedness, etc. They may not be able to speak to you if they have a mouthpiece in place, so it will help greatly if you ask yes or no questions or questions that can be answered with a thumbs-up or thumbs-down. Any signs suggestive of confusion or near-syncope are obvious reasons to discontinue the test.

It is particularly important to obtain some sense of whether the patient gave a full effort. In most cases, this will not be an issue, but there will be an occasional patient who quits early or otherwise does not give a full effort and the data are less helpful. The best clues to whether or not they gave a full effort are what they look like at the end of the test. Diaphoresis and marked tachypnea as well as the presence of a ventilatory threshold in the data all suggest that the patient gave a full effort. Finally, to help ensure that they give a full effort, one of your jobs is to be a cheerleader and to push them on when they do not feel like doing so. As long as there are no significant ECG abnormalities, blood pressure does not decrease, and the individual remains alert, patients should be encouraged to continue exercising. A $\dot{V}O_{2\,max}$ can only be determined from a maximum effort.

STOPPING THE TEST
We strive to have people pedal at 60–70 rpm and have them continue this cadence until they reach exhaustion and cannot maintain that pedal rate, despite encouragement. The cardiopulmonary exercise test is a symptom-limited test and, in most cases, we do not stop the test because people reach a threshold value for certain parameters,

such as their heart rate. In most cases, the end-point of the test is easy to identify. For normal patients or patients with cardiac limitation this point comes when their legs become tired and they can no longer turn the pedals. For patients with ventilatory limitation this point comes when they become too short of breath. For the ventilatory limitation patients, you can often anticipate when this will happen by comparing their actual minute ventilation with their pretest maximum voluntary ventilation (MVV). As the former approaches the latter, they will typically become too short of breath to continue and will soon be signaling you that they need to stop.

There are, however, specific indications for you to stop the exercise test before the subject reaches exhaustion. These indications include: [1]

- Significant arrhythmia (short bursts of ventricular tachycardia, sustained ventricular tachycardia)
- Second- or third-degree heart block
- Failure to maintain systolic blood pressure (i.e., any decrease) during heavy exercise
- ST segment depression ≥ 2 mm
- Patient distress
- Chest pain suggestive of cardiac ischemia
- Loss of coordination
- Near-syncope, dizziness, or confusion
- Symptomatic severe hypoxemia ($SpO_2 < 80\%$)

When the patient reaches exhaustion and asks to stop exercising, the resistance is removed from the bicycle or the speed of the treadmill is decreased and the grade flattened. It is very important that the patient continue pedaling without resistance or walking slowly on the flat to maintain venous return to the heart and, as a result, maintain cardiac output at levels sufficient to perfuse the central nervous system and prevent syncope. They should also remain connected to the monitoring equipment, as important data are collected during this period.

ADDITIONAL CONCERNS WITH CARDIAC DISEASE PATIENTS

There are two additional issues of which you should be aware when exercising patients with known cardiomyopathy or coronary artery disease. First, questions arise about when to stop the test in patients with known coronary artery disease. As noted earlier, ECG monitoring is performed throughout the test and the ECGs should be reviewed during and after the test for evidence of ischemia. However, if a patient has left bundle branch block at baseline, the exercise ECG will not be useful for this purpose. One useful change in the ECG pattern, however, would be the new onset of a left bundle branch block. Because of this problem, when you exercise a patient with known or possible coronary artery disease and an abnormal baseline ECG, you should be especially vigilant about monitoring the exercise blood pressures. As noted above, we generally stop tests based on symptoms alone, and not because people reach a particular threshold for any one parameter such as age-predicted maximum heart rate. Either an abnormal blood pressure response or a progressive pattern of ventricular premature contractions at higher exercise levels represents reasons for the physician to stop the test.

Second, you must have a heightened awareness for the possibility of ventricular arrhythmia. In general, the worst arrhythmias are seen during the post-exertional (recovery) phase of the test. The incidence of such arrhythmias in our lab appears to have decreased with the now routine use of beta-blockers in this population. Even in patients on adequate beta-blocker regimens, however, it is still important to remain vigilant about the possibility of arrhythmias during and after the test.

AFTER THE TEST IS COMPLETED

IMMEDIATELY FOLLOWING THE TEST

As noted above, when the test is complete, the patient must continue pedaling (unloaded/no resistance) or walking slowly on a flat incline in order to prevent syncope. Data should continue to be collected during this recovery period, including at least two additional blood pressure measurements, as this information can aid in determining the degree of exercise dysfunction (see below). Young, unfit subjects who have given a true maximum effort may have a postexercise vagal response and should keep pedaling or walking with very frequent blood pressure checks. If they do not maintain acceptable systolic pressures, they should be immediately taken off the bicycle and kept supine with legs elevated. If any postexercise patient manifest confusion and/or cannot continue pedaling, they must be helped off the bicycle or treadmill and kept supine for at least 10 minute with intermittent blood pressure and continuous ECG monitoring. If they remain symptomatic at that point, further medical evaluation may be warranted.

TAKING THE PATIENT OFF THE CYCLE ERGOMETER OR TREADMILL

After the patient has adequately cooled down, they can be disconnected from the equipment and allowed to take a seat. It is fine to give them some water at this point. You should observe them for a few minutes to ensure that they have no further issues (e.g., arrhythmia). As noted above, the worst ventricular arrhythmias actually tend to occur in the post-exertional phase of the test.

Some patients will ask you how they did on the test. The data from an exercise test can usually be printed out immediately, thereby allowing you to provide some feedback to them about their performance. However, adequate interpretation of the data often requires a thorough review of the data, so you should be measured in the conclusions you provide to the patient in the period immediately following the test.

ASK THE PATIENT WHY THEY STOPPED AT THE END OF THE TEST

Before the testing session is completed, it is important to ask the patient why they had to stop cycling or walking/running at the end the test, as the answer is an important part of test interpretation. As noted above and in Chap. 3, patients with cardiac limitation tend to stop because of leg fatigue, while patients with ventilatory limitation usually stop because they are out of breath. Patients may occasionally give other responses, such as the fact that they were having severe joint pain, but more often than not they will say that they stopped due to leg fatigue or dyspnea.

In addition to inquiring as to why they stopped the test, it is worthwhile to ask if they had other important symptoms such as chest pain or lightheadedness or whether the symptoms they felt on the bicycle are similar to the symptoms that limit their ability to exert themselves in their daily lives.

RESET IMPLANTED DEFIBRILLATORS BACK TO ORIGINAL SETTINGS

If a patient has an implantable defibrillator or pacemaker and the settings were changed for the purpose of the test, the settings should be changed back to their original values prior to the patient leaving the exercise-testing laboratory.

WHAT HAPPENS NEXT

Once the test is completed and the patient leaves the testing laboratory, the next task will be to interpret the test results. The method for doing this and an example of a cardiopulmonary exercise test report from our laboratory are provided in the next chapter.

CYCLE ERGOMETRY VERSUS TREADMILL

As noted above and elsewhere in this primer, cardiopulmonary exercise tests can be performed using either cycle ergometers or treadmills. This fact often leads to questions as to which is the superior modality for conducting the studies. One important difference between the modalities is that individuals generally achieve modestly higher maximum oxygen uptake on the treadmill than on a cycle ergometer [2, 7]. The differences are generally small, however, and, as a result, likely not of great clinical significance. Other advantages and disadvantages of the two testing modalities are described in Table 4.2.

Each diagnostics laboratory will have its preferred method for conducting cardiopulmonary exercise tests. At our institution, for example, the preferred method is cycle ergometry. Even though there may be a preferred method, however, it is helpful to have both an ergometer and treadmill available for tests and for the individuals conducting and interpreting tests be familiar with both modalities as certain patient factors may preclude the use of a particular method.

TABLE 4.2 ADVANTAGES AND DISADVANTAGES OF CYCLE ERGOMETRY AND TREADMILL TESTING

Cycle ergometry	
Advantages	**Disadvantages**
Permits assessment of power output	Patients achieve about 10% lower $\dot{V}O_{2\,max}$ compared to the treadmill
Patient can stop exercise without assistance from the test supervisor	Patients may be unfamiliar with pedaling a bicycle
Safer for patients with coordination problems or risk of syncope	
Fewer artifacts in ventilatory, blood pressure, and circulatory measurements	
Easier to obtain blood gas samples	
Treadmill	
Advantages	**Disadvantages**
Patients achieve higher $\dot{V}O_{2\,max}$ compared to the cycle ergometer	Difficult to quantify the work rate
Familiarity of exercise for patients that more closely approximates activities of daily living	The patient's ability to stop exercising is dependent on the ability of the test supervisor to respond to their request

REFERENCES

1. American Thoracic Society, American College of Chest Physicians. ATS/ACCP statement on cardiopulmonary exercise testing. Am J Respir Crit Care Med. 2003;167(2):211–77.
2. Wasserman K, Hansen JE, Sue DY, Stringer WW, Whipp BJ. Principles of exercise testing and interpretation. 4th ed. Philadelphia: Lippincott, Williams and Wilkins; 2005.
3. Jones NL. Clinical exercise testing. 4th ed. Philadelphia: Saunders; 1997.
4. Nagle FJ, Balke B, Naughton JP. Gradational step tests for assessing work capacity. J Appl Physiol. 1965;20:745–8.
5. Bruce RA. Exercise testing of patients with coronary artery disease. Principles and normal standards for evaluation. Ann Clin Res. 1971;3:323–32.
6. Porszasz J, Casaburi R, Somfay A, Woodhouse L, Whipp B. A treadmill ramp protocol using simultaneous changes in speed and grade. Med Sci Sports Exerc. 2003;35:1596–603.
7. Hansen JE. Exercise instruments, schemes and protocols for evaluating the dyspneic patient. Am Rev Respir Dis. 1984;129(suppl):S25–7.

Chapter 5
Interpreting the Results of Cardiopulmonary Exercise Tests

Keywords Anaerobic threshold • Carbon dioxide production • Cardiac limitation • Cardiac output • Dead space fraction • Diaphoresis • End-tidal carbon dioxide • End-tidal oxygen • Forced expiratory volume in one second • Forced vital capacity • Heart rate reserve • Interstitial lung disease • Lactate threshold • Maximum oxygen consumption • Maximum voluntary ventilation • Metabolic acidosis • Minute ventilation • Oxygen consumption • Oxygen pulse (O_2 pulse) • Oxygen saturation • Power • Pulmonary vascular disease • Respiratory exchange ratio • Tidal volume • Troubleshooting • Ventilation • Ventilatory equivalents for carbon dioxide • Ventilatory equivalents for oxygen • Ventilatory limitation • Ventilatory reserve • Ventilatory threshold • V-Slope method

INTERPRETING CARDIOPULMONARY EXERCISE TESTS

Once the data collection portion of the cardiopulmonary exercise test has been completed, the final task is to interpret the results of the test. This section of the primer provides general information regarding test interpretation as well as suggestions for the content and format of the final report. It also reviews one of the key components of test interpretation—identification of the ventilatory threshold.

A.M. Luks et al., *Introduction to Cardiopulmonary Exercise Testing*, DOI 10.1007/978-1-4614-6283-5_5, © Springer Science+Business Media New York 2013

TROUBLESHOOTING THE DATA

Before starting data interpretation and your report, you should do some basic troubleshooting of the data to ensure that there are no systematic errors that may affect data interpretation. The primary troubleshooting steps include the following:

Step 1: *Check the* $\dot{V}O_2$ *at rest and during unloaded pedaling*. At rest, the $\dot{V}O_2$ should be around 250 ml/minute for a normal-sized person. During unloaded pedaling, you should expect to see a value around 400 ml/minute. In obese individuals, both the resting and unloaded pedaling values will be higher (e.g., 1,000 ml/minute with unloaded pedaling).

Step 2: *Check the respiratory exchange ratio* (R). R should remain between 0.8 and 0.95 for the first 30–40% of the test before rising thereafter. It should never be below 0.7. If the patient gave a good maximal effort, R tends to rise to between 1.1 and 1.3 at peak exercise and should continue to rise for 1–2 minutes after the test is complete as carbon dioxide stores wash out but oxygen consumption declines. Individuals may hyperventilate at rest or in early exercise, resulting in an $R > 1.0$. If this is observed, you should extend the rest period or unloaded pedaling until R decreases toward a normal value. Abnormal R values usually suggest problems with the oxygen sensor, but you should also consider mask leaks or problems with the sampling catheter.

Step 3: *Check the relationship between oxygen consumption and watts expended*. Once the subject begins loaded pedaling, oxygen consumption as a function of work should increase in a linear and predictable manner; oxygen consumption should increase at roughly 10 ml O_2/W on the cycle ergometer. Smaller rates of increase usually suggest that the rate of watt increase (the ramp) was too steep for the subject.

Step 4: *Check the oxygen saturation data*. If you notice that the oxygen saturation fell during the test, you need to decide if this was a true result. Subjects who truly desaturate do so in a steady, progressive manner with the lowest numbers observed in the first minute after the bicycle load is removed or treadmill is slowed down. The oxygen saturation also returns to baseline slowly, often over 1–2 minutes. When there are problems with sensor placement or poor signal, the oxygen saturation data will be more chaotic and will not follow a clear trend.

Step 5: *Check for leaks in the system*. In the past, we have struggled with gas leaks from the mask or other connections in the system that give distorted data. Clues to the presence of this problem include a very early plateau in $\dot{V}O_2$ (i.e., $\dot{V}O_2$ fails to rise as work rate continues to rise for more than a 1–2-minutes period), inappropriate R-values, and inappropriately high $P_{ET}O_2$ values.

Once you have gone through these steps and ensured that there are no systematic errors, you are ready to interpret the data and create your report. If a systematic error was identified, it is important to work with the technician who helped perform the test to identify the source of the problem and correct it, if possible. In some cases, the test may need to be repeated in order to obtain the information necessary to answer the clinical question.

IDENTIFYING THE VENTILATORY THRESHOLD

The term "ventilatory threshold" refers to an important point in a cardiopulmonary exercise test where a number of ventilatory parameters exhibit a threshold-like response during progressive exercise. It is temporally related to the development of a lactic acidosis. Other terms for this transition timepoint include "lactate threshold" or "anaerobic threshold." At our institution we prefer to use the term "ventilatory threshold" because serum lactate levels are not measured in many cardiopulmonary exercise tests. Although the term was originally thought to represent the development of muscle hypoxia in the late stages of exercise, it turns out that lactate levels rise as a result of a more complex process than simply anaerobic metabolism. While opinions differ on the functional significance of events in muscle leading to lactic acidosis, the ventilatory threshold may identify a level of exertion where blood flow to the exercising muscle is no longer able to completely meet the metabolic demands.

Identification of the ventilatory threshold is a critical step in cardiopulmonary exercise test interpretation to identify the organ system limiting exercise. Therefore, before describing other aspects of cardiopulmonary exercise test interpretation and how to document the results in a report, we will describe methods by which to determine whether the threshold is present and address several important issues associated with this concept.

WHY THE VENTILATORY THRESHOLD IS IMPORTANT IN EXERCISE TESTING

As noted above, the ventilatory threshold is a point during a progressive work exercise test where a number of ventilatory parameters demonstrate a threshold-like response and is indicative of the point where blood flow of the exercising muscles is no longer sufficient to meet its metabolic demand. Ventilatory thresholds are typically not seen in individuals who stop exercising before reaching this presumed perfusion limitation to exercising muscle (i.e., patients who stop because of respiratory or muscle problems). Given this important difference between these underlying disease processes, we can use the presence or the absence of the ventilatory threshold as an important criterion in our effort to identify the cause of exercise limitation in a given patient.

WHEN DOES THE VENTILATORY THRESHOLD OCCUR DURING EXERCISE

In most untrained, healthy individuals, the anaerobic threshold occurs at about 50–65% of maximum oxygen uptake ($\dot{V}O_{2\,max}$) while in very fit and elderly individuals it may occur at a greater percentage of the $\dot{V}O_{2\,max}$.

For most of the studies you will interpret, the precise time point at which the threshold occurs is not as important as whether or not it is present. In fact, the ventilatory threshold is probably better viewed as a "zone" rather than a distinct point in the exercise period.

In research studies or exercise training programs, identifying the precise point at which the ventilatory threshold occurs may be more important than in cardiopulmonary exercise tests used for diagnostic purposes. In exercise training programs for elite athletes, for example, the goal may be to have the athlete perform steady-state exercise at their ventilatory threshold for a defined period of time. In such cases, it would be important to know the specific $\dot{V}O_2$ and level of power output at which the threshold was present.

GRAPHICAL METHODS FOR IDENTIFYING THE VENTILATORY THRESHOLD

There are several methods by which the ventilatory threshold can be identified and it is useful to be familiar with each of these techniques. Rather than relying on a single method during test interpretation, a more robust approach is to confirm the presence or the absence of the ventilatory threshold by examining the data using several of the methods described below.

The V-Slope Method

Before the ventilatory threshold is reached, $\dot{V}O_2$ and $\dot{V}CO_2$ increase at steady rates. Once the ventilatory threshold is reached and a metabolic acidosis develops, the rate of rise in $\dot{V}CO_2$ will exceed that of $\dot{V}O_2$. This changing relationship can be used to identify the ventilatory threshold using a technique known as the "V-slope" method. $\dot{V}CO_2$ is plotted against $\dot{V}O_2$, with the former on the y-axis and the latter on the x-axis (Fig. 5.1). This plot is typically the middle graph in the 9-box plot described in Chap. 3 (Fig. 3.1e). As noted above, the two

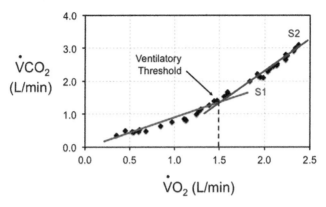

Fig. 5.1 The V-slope method for identifying the ventilatory threshold. Before the threshold, $\dot{V}CO_2$ and $\dot{V}O_2$ rise at roughly the same rate. The best-fit line through these points is labeled S1 and is denoted with *red color*. After the threshold, $\dot{V}CO_2$ rises faster than $\dot{V}O_2$. The best-fit line through these points is labeled S2 and is denoted with *blue color*. The point at which S1 and S2 intersect represents the ventilatory threshold

variables will rise at a steady rate before the ventilatory threshold and a best-fit line through these points will have a slope close to R. Once the ventilatory threshold is reached, the $\dot{V}CO_2$ will rise at a much faster rate. In fact, two different slopes can often be identified due to temporal differences in the metabolic and respiratory compensations for increasing carbon dioxide production. A second best-fit line through the points will now have a greater slope. The point at which the two best-fit lines intersect is the ventilatory threshold. This method is the classic method described by Wasserman and colleagues in their text on cardiopulmonary exercise testing [1]. The clarity of this break-point and, therefore, the certainty of the ventilatory threshold vary across individuals. It is most prominent in individuals with strong ventilatory drives and less obvious in elderly individuals and individuals taking beta-blockers for management of cardiomyopathy.

Changes in Minute Ventilation
Minute ventilation rises throughout exercise until the subject reaches the ventilatory threshold, after which the rate of rise of minute ventilation increases appreciably. As a result, if you follow the plot of $\dot{V}E$ versus $\dot{V}CO_2$ (Fig. 5.2), you will see a change in the slope of this relationship. A similar change in slope can be identified in a plot of $\dot{V}E$ versus work rate. This relative increase in minute ventilation comes later than the ventilatory threshold identified by the V-slope method described above.

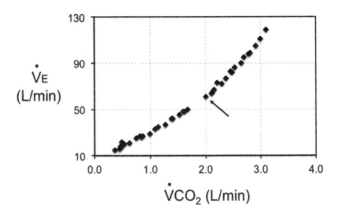

Fig. 5.2 $\dot{V}_E$ versus $\dot{V}CO_2$ as a means for identifying whether a ventilatory threshold is present. The *black arrow* denotes a point at which there is a change in the slope of the relationship between $\dot{V}_E$ and $\dot{V}CO_2$. This inflection point occurs around the time of the ventilatory threshold

Changes in Ventilatory Equivalents

Once a subject reaches their ventilatory threshold, the ventilatory equivalents for both oxygen ($\dot{V}_E/\dot{V}O_2$) and carbon dioxide ($\dot{V}_E/\dot{V}CO_2$), which generally remain stable through the early part of exercise, start a steady rise (Fig. 5.3), with the increase in $\dot{V}_E/\dot{V}O_2$ coming before the $\dot{V}_E/\dot{V}CO_2$. The ventilatory threshold is identified at the increase in the ventilatory equivalent for oxygen, not at the increase in the ventilatory equivalent for carbon dioxide.

Changes in End-Tidal Oxygen and Carbon Dioxide Tensions

In addition to affecting the ventilatory equivalents, the increase in minute ventilation out of proportion to oxygen consumption and carbon dioxide production will also cause alveolar oxygen tensions to increase and carbon dioxide tensions to decrease. As a result, in the graphical plots of these data points you will see an increase in end-tidal oxygen levels ($P_{ET}O_2$), a surrogate measure of alveolar oxygen tension, and a decrease in end-total carbon dioxide levels ($P_{ET}CO_2$), a surrogate measure for the alveolar carbon dioxide tension. Again, the increase in $P_{ET}O_2$ will precede the decrease in $P_{ET}CO_2$ (Fig. 5.4).

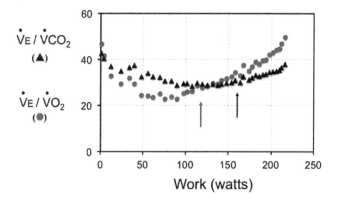

Fig. 5.3 Using changes in ventilatory equivalents as a means to identify whether a ventilatory threshold is present. Because minute ventilation increases at the ventilatory threshold, the $\dot{V}E/\dot{V}CO_2$ (*black*) and $\dot{V}E/\dot{V}O_2$ (*red*) begin a steady rise. The point at which $\dot{V}E/\dot{V}CO_2$ starts to rise is denoted by a *black arrow* while the point at which $\dot{V}E/\dot{V}O_2$ starts to rise is denoted by a *red arrow*. Note that $\dot{V}E/\dot{V}O_2$ starts to rise earlier than $\dot{V}E/\dot{V}CO_2$, a commonly seen pattern in individuals with a cardiac limitation pattern, including normal individuals. The point where the ventilatory equivalent for oxygen begins to increase is a marker for the ventilatory threshold. The ventilatory equivalent for carbon dioxide begins to rise after the ventilatory threshold

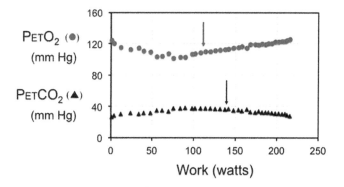

Fig. 5.4 Using changes in end-tidal oxygen and carbon dioxide tensions as a means to identify whether a ventilatory threshold is present. Because minute ventilation increases out of proportion to oxygen consumption and carbon dioxide production at the ventilatory threshold, end-tidal oxygen tensions (*red*) begin a steady rise while end-tidal carbon dioxide tensions (*black*) begin a steady fall somewhat later in exercise. The point at which $P_{ET}O_2$ begins to rise is denoted by the *red arrow* while the point at which $P_{ET}CO_2$ begins to decrease is denoted by the *black arrow*

USING THE RAW DATA TO IDENTIFY THE VENTILATORY THRESHOLD

The methods of identifying the ventilatory threshold described above all involve using graphs from the 9-box plot that accompanies the data output from most cardiopulmonary exercise testing systems. In addition to examining these graphical displays, it is also possible to examine the printed sequence of numerical data to identify the ventilatory threshold. An example of the raw data output is provided in Fig. 5.5. Arrows have been added to the data columns to identify where variables start changing in patterns consistent with those seen at the ventilatory threshold. $P_{ET}O_2$, $\dot{V}_E/\dot{V}CO_2$, and $\dot{V}_E/\dot{V}O_2$ begin a steeper, steady rise while $P_{ET}CO_2$ decreases. Note that each variable does not start changing at precisely the same time. There will be some differences in the break points for each variable. The important feature is that these break points are present, indicating that the patient has a ventilatory threshold. The precise position of that threshold will be in the general vicinity of all of these break points.

ARTERIAL BLOOD GASES

As mentioned above, one of the key aspects of the ventilatory threshold is the temporal association with the development of a lactic acidosis. If arterial blood gases are obtained on an exercising subject, you can easily identify whether or not a ventilatory threshold is present by reviewing the blood gases and identifying when the bicarbonate value begins to fall from its baseline and the $PaCO_2$ falls. In addition, depending on the blood gas analyzer, serum lactate levels can also be measured from the blood gas sample. The downside of this method is that blood gases are drawn at intervals and, as a result, may not help you identify precisely when the threshold was reached. Because the majority of the subjects who undergo cardiopulmonary exercise testing do not have arterial lines placed for their test, this method is not always available.

BLOOD PRESSURE AND DIAPHORESIS

Catecholamine levels increase significantly around the same time as the ventilatory threshold. It is therefore common to observe a stepwise increase in the systolic blood pressure at the same time as the ventilatory threshold. Subjects begin to sweat about this same time. These physical observations can increase the confidence in the presence of a ventilatory threshold among subjects who give a maximal effort.

Work (Watts)	VO₂ (L/min)	VCO₂ (L/min)	VE (L/min)	HR (bpm)	R	VE/VO₂	VE/VCO₂	PETO₂ (mmHg)	PETCO₂ (mmHg)
1	0.45	0.49	22	90	1.09	47	43	125	27
4	0.35	0.36	15	88	1.03	42	40	121	29
12	0.53	0.47	18	89	0.89	33	37	115	31
24	0.54	0.45	16	96	0.84	29	35	112	32
34	0.61	0.53	20	96	0.87	32	37	115	31
40	0.60	0.47	18	98	0.79	29	37	111	32
48	0.84	0.63	21	106	0.75	24	32	109	32
56	0.68	0.48	17	104	0.70	24	34	103	35
62	1.13	0.81	27	113	0.72	24	33	104	35
70	0.97	0.75	25	116	0.77	25	32	108	34
76	1.13	0.84	26	115	0.75	23	31	102	38
84	1.11	0.86	27	120	0.77	24	31	103	38
90	1.25	0.99	29	126	0.79	23	29	103	38
98	1.27	1.09	33	132	0.86	25	30	107	38
102	1.29	1.14	35	134	0.88	26	30	108	38
108	1.39	1.27	37	138	0.91	26	29	109	38
114	1.45	1.39	42	142	0.96	29	30	110	37
120	1.47	1.40	42	144	0.95	28	29	110 ←	38
126	1.55	1.53	45	150	0.99	28	29	111 ←	37
132	1.59	1.59	48	153	1.00	30	29	112	37
138	1.60	1.62	48	155	1.02	29	29	112	37
142	1.59	1.68	50	156	1.06	31 ←	29 ←	113	37
148	1.99	2.11	64	162	1.06	32	30 ←	115	35 ←
154	1.84	2.00	61	167	1.09	33	30	115	36
158	1.93	2.15	67	167	1.11	34	31	117	35
164	1.95	2.13	65	171	1.09	33	30	115	36
168	1.92	2.21	73	171	1.15	37	32	119	33
174	2.04	2.29	72	173	1.12	35	31	119	33
178	2.06	2.37	77	179	1.15	37	32	118	34
182	2.10	2.45	83	180	1.17	39	33	120	32
186	2.14	2.48	82	182	1.16	38	33	119	33
190	2.14	2.53	86	182	1.18	40	33	120	32
194	2.23	2.65	90	184	1.18	40	34	121	32
198	2.22	2.70	95	184	1.22	42	35	122	31
202	2.25	2.78	98	184	1.24	43	35	122	31
206	2.23	2.81	99	186	1.26	44	35	123	31
210	2.32	2.91	105	186	1.25	45	36	123	30
212	2.34	3.00	111	189	1.28	47	37	125	29
216	2.38	3.10	119	186	1.30	50	38	126	28

Fig. 5.5 Analyzing the printed sequence of numerical data from a cardiopulmonary exercise test to identify the ventilatory threshold. *Red arrows* have been added to the display to indicate the approximate locations where $P_{ET}O_2$, $P_{ET}CO_2$, $\dot{V}E/\dot{V}CO_2$, and $\dot{V}E/\dot{V}CO_2$ start to change in patterns consistent with those seen at the ventilatory threshold. $P_{ET}O_2$, $\dot{V}E/\dot{V}O_2$, and $\dot{V}E/\dot{V}CO_2$ begin a steeper, steady rise while $P_{ET}CO_2$ decreases. These data were taken from the same test used to generate Figs. 5.1–5.4

OTHER ISSUES PERTAINING TO THE VENTILATORY THRESHOLD

In the course of interpreting cardiopulmonary exercise tests, several questions often arise regarding the ventilatory threshold that are useful to consider in greater detail.

Does the precise location of the threshold matter? All reviewers may not agree on the exact location of the ventilatory threshold, but generally agree on whether it is present or absent. As noted earlier, for the majority of tests you will do, the key question is whether or not it is present. The exact point at which it occurs rarely changes the interpretation of the test. There are cases where knowing the precise location of the threshold is important, however. As noted earlier, this can be important in research studies or exercise training protocols. In addition, it may be important to determine if there is a change in the onset of the ventilatory threshold following an intervention in a given patient.

Will I always see a ventilatory threshold? As noted above, patients with obstructive lung disease may lack a ventilatory threshold if they stop because their ventilatory pump fails before the heart reaches the limit of its ability to generate cardiac output. Patients with cardiac limitation (e.g., cardiomyopathy) on the other hand generally have an identifiable ventilatory threshold. You should be aware, however, that a significant proportion of cardiomyopathy patients will be on beta-blockers as part of their treatment regimen and our experience in the laboratory has been that the presence of beta-blockers sometimes makes it difficult for us to identify a clear ventilatory threshold. They certainly help prevent ventricular tachycardia during the testing but also make the data interpretation difficult at times. Elderly subjects can have delayed onset of a ventilatory threshold, sometimes to the point of not even having an identifiable threshold.

Can you develop a lactic acidosis and not see an increase in minute ventilation? It is possible for this to occur. Patients with severe chronic obstructive pulmonary disease may develop a lactic acidosis but may not be able to increase their minute ventilation adequately to compensate for this process. You might notice this problem when analyzing the arterial blood gas data, in which case you would see a progressive metabolic acidosis but no compensatory fall in the $PaCO_2$. What matters most from a clinical standpoint, however, is the failure to mount a ventilatory response. Whether or not a patient develops a lactic acidosis, the failure to mount a ventilatory response is indicative of ventilatory limitation as the likely source of the patient's exercise limitation. You do not need to put an arterial line in all individuals to tease out whether they had a lactic acidosis in addition to their ventilatory limitation as this is unlikely to alter your test interpretation or recommendations to the requesting provider.

INTERPRETING THE DATA AND CREATING YOUR REPORT

The process of interpreting the data and reporting the results will be easier if it is broken up into discrete blocks that become separate sections in the report. Each of the blocks is described in detail below. A sample report from our laboratory is provided in the Appendix to this chapter.

The specific details of the report may vary from institution to institution and the learner is encouraged to discuss the specific format with their supervisor as they go about the test interpretation and reporting process.

INDICATIONS FOR THE TEST AND OTHER RELEVANT CLINICAL DATA

We suggest you begin your report with a short paragraph in which you review the primary reasons for performing the test. In this section, you should also note the patient's age, gender, height, and weight; whether the patient is on any relevant cardiac or pulmonary medications such as beta-blockers; and whether they have undergone any cardiac or thoracic surgical procedures.

PULMONARY FUNCTION TEST RESULTS

Patients perform spirometry prior to starting the exercise test to document their FEV_1, FVC, FEV_1/FVC, and their maximum voluntary ventilation (MVV), important data points that will be used in the interpretation of the test results. The results of the spirometry testing as well as an interpretation of these results should be added to the report.

FACTORS LIMITING EXERCISE

Document the work increment used (e.g., 10 W/minute ramp), and the maximum power attained. If the subject was tested on a treadmill, describe the treadmill protocol that was chosen and the time and stage when the subject had to stop. Specify the subject's stated reason for stopping the test: Did they stop because of leg fatigue, dyspnea, chest pain, or lightheadedness? You should also document whether the exercise-limiting symptoms during the test duplicated the exertional symptoms they have at home.

In your report, you should also note whether the patient gave a full effort. You will have a sense of this by looking at the patient at the end of exercise (sweating, clearly working hard) but the best sign will be if the patient exercised past a ventilatory threshold (although you should remember that people with ventilatory limitation will not generally reach one). Maximal exercise heart rate is not a good indicator of whether someone gave a full effort because of the wide range of maximal exercise heart rates in normal individuals and hence an inability to accurately predict an individual's maximum heart rate. In addition, many test subjects will be on beta-blockers and their heart rates will not rise as they would in individuals not on these medications. Similarly, the respiratory quotient, R, is not a reliable predictor of maximal effort, as an individual with respiratory limitation may not reach a ventilatory threshold. In general, relying on one variable to determine whether the test subject gave a good effort is less reliable and the use of multiple factors provides a more robust determination of effort.

MAXIMAL OXYGEN CONSUMPTION

In this section, you should note the maximum oxygen consumption ($\dot{V}O_{2\,max}$) and how this compares to the predicted values. Most exercise systems base their predicted values on age, gender, and weight. Weight-based predictions are likely most appropriate if a person's weight is primarily muscle. However, obese individuals have relatively less muscle per weight and weight-based predictions of oxygen consumptions are less valuable in these subjects. In our laboratory, we therefore use Jones' predictions [2], which are height- rather than weight-based predictions for oxygen consumption. You should report the values in ml/minute as well as the weight-normalized values. We also report maximum oxygen consumption per ideal body weight ($\dot{V}O_{2\,max}$/IBW) to demonstrate what the weight-normalized oxygen consumption would be if the subject were not obese. Due to the populations from which the Jones-predicted values were derived, some of our calculated normal values may not be appropriate for people under the age of 20. There are also poor data for the elderly, especially elderly

TABLE 5.1 NORMAL VALUES FOR TEST PARAMETERS

Parameter	Range
$(A-a)\Delta O_2$ (mmHg)	Rest: 5–20 (the upper limit of normal increases with age)
Maximum heart rate (bpm)	Predicted = 220 – age or 210 – (0.65 × age), Normal: 90% predicted ± 15 bpm
Maximum V_T (l)	About 60% of the forced vital capacity
$\dot{V}_E$ (l/min)	Peak exercise: <60–80% of the measured maximum voluntary ventilation
O_2 pulse (ml/beat)	Predicted: (Predicted $\dot{V}O_{2\,max}$)/(predicted max HR) Normal: >80% predicted (~15 ml/beat in men; ~10 ml/beat in women)
$P_{ET}CO_2$ (mmHg)	35–42 (should decline to lower values after ventilatory threshold)
$P_{ET}O_2$ (mmHg)	100–115 (should rise to higher values after ventilatory threshold)
Respiratory exchange ratio	Rest: 0.7–0.85, peak exercise: 1.1–1.3[a]
SaO_2 (%)	≥95% (should remain constant with exercise)
V_D/V_T	0.25–0.35 at rest (should decrease with exercise)
$\dot{V}_E/\dot{V}CO_2$ (early exercise)	24–34
$\dot{V}_E/\dot{V}O_2$ (early exercise)	22–32
$\dot{V}O_{2\,max}$ (ml/min)	>80% predicted for the test subject based on gender, age, and height
$\dot{V}O_{2\,rest}$ (ml/min)	Normal: 200–350 (depending on size)

[a]Increases in the respiratory exchange ratio >1.3 can be seen in patients with a cardiac limitation pattern, especially during the recovery phase

women. A table of normal values for this and many other key parameters is provided in Table 5.1.

When considering the maximum oxygen consumption, an important point to remember is that a subject's $\dot{V}O_{2\,max}$ may fall within the "normal" range or even exceed the predicted values, yet that person may still have experienced a loss of exercise capacity compared to their prior baseline. To illustrate this point, consider the case of an elite rower we saw in our laboratory several years ago. After a long plane flight, he developed increased dyspnea on exertion and could no longer keep up with his teammates at practice. He did a cardiopulmonary exercise test and achieved a $\dot{V}O_{2\,max}$ of over 60 ml/kg/minute. That number was well above his predicted value and on the surface appeared "normal." However, it is likely that had we tested him prior to his plane flight, the $\dot{V}O_{2\,max}$ might have been 75 ml/kg/minute. He could clearly tell us that something was different and the 60 ml/kg/minute value was not "normal" for him. It turned out that he experienced a pulmonary embolism on his plane flight and now had pulmonary vascular limitation to exercise.

Whether or not the subject is obese will also affect your interpretation of maximum exercise capacity. "Normal" obese subjects all should have maximal oxygen consumption at or above a height-predicted (i.e., IBW) normal value.

THE CARDIOVASCULAR RESPONSE

You should begin this section by noting the resting and maximal heart rate attained and the resting rhythm. You should also review the ECG tracings, looking for ST segment changes or arrhythmias and when in the progression of the test they were observed. Describe the blood pressure response to exercise. It should rise progressively with exercise, with the largest increases seen after the ventilatory threshold. A falling blood pressure during heavy exercise, as noted in other sections of this primer, suggests significant heart disease, and is an indication to immediately terminate the test. Note the changes in the O_2 pulse, a surrogate marker for stroke volume. This should rise progressively through exercise and plateau once the patient achieves their $\dot{V}O_{2\,max}$. Finally, identify whether or not a ventilatory threshold was present. This last step, described in detail above, is a key part of interpreting the primary cause of a patient's exercise limitation. You should note the point at which it occurred relative to the $\dot{V}O_{2\,max}$. In most individuals, this will occur at about 60% of the $\dot{V}O_{2\,max}$ while in highly trained endurance athletes, it may occur at 80% of their maximum exercise capacity. The ventilatory threshold comes later with age and active patients over the age of 80 may show a threshold either very late in exercise or not at all.

VENTILATORY RESPONSE

The goal in this part of the interpretation is to identify whether the patient has any evidence of ventilatory limitation. After noting the peak respiratory rate and the maximum tidal volume achieved, compare the maximum minute ventilation at peak exercise with the MVV. In patients with ventilatory limitation, the minute ventilation at peak exercise will be much closer to their MVV. Subjects without pulmonary abnormalities will have a maximal exercise ventilation less than 80% of their MVV, although a few very fit athletes are capable of raising their minute ventilation close to their MVV. The other important indication of a ventilatory limitation is $PETCO_2$ that fails to decrease during the last minutes of a maximal effort.

You should also examine the ventilatory equivalents for carbon dioxide and oxygen, as these values are reflective of alveolar ventilation. Normal $\dot{V}E/\dot{V}CO_2$ values should be about 24–34 at lower levels of exercise below the ventilatory threshold and rise to higher levels once a subject passes their ventilatory threshold. Values lower than this suggest an intrinsically blunted ventilatory drive, while higher values indicate alveolar hyperventilation and/or increased dead space. Be aware that many patients and normal subjects get "amped up" when they get on the bicycle and hyperventilate while sitting at rest or during unloaded pedaling. They will demonstrate elevated ventilatory equivalents as a result of this but the values tend to come back down to normal levels once they begin loaded pedaling.

GAS EXCHANGE AND BLOOD GASES

In this section, you should note the trends in end-tidal oxygen and carbon dioxide and whether or not there were changes in oxygen saturation. Oxygen saturation should remain constant in normal individuals and patients with cardiac limitation, whereas it may fall in patients with obstructive, pulmonary vascular or interstitial lung disease, or intracardiac shunts. $P_{ET}O_2$ typically rises once the subject has passed their ventilatory threshold. $P_{ET}CO_2$ will fall after patients reach their ventilatory threshold but will increase or remain stable in patients with ventilatory limitation.

You will not have blood gases in every patient. If you do obtain them, it is helpful to present the data from all of the blood gas measurements in a table. You should also note the alveolar-arterial oxygen difference $[(A-a)\Delta O_2]$. In calculating the alveolar PO_2 to determine the $(A-a)\Delta O_2$, remember to use the R from the exercise study at the time the arterial blood gas was obtained. The $(A-a)\Delta O_2$ should remain within the range of age-predicted normal values at rest and through moderate levels of exercise before widening at end-exercise. There are no data describing the normal $(A-a)\Delta O_2$ across different age groups at maximum exercise.

You should then identify changes in the bicarbonate and the $PaCO_2$. The bicarbonate starts to fall around the ventilatory threshold and the $PaCO_2$ should drop progressively in response to this metabolic acidosis. A stable or increasing $PaCO_2$ is evidence of ventilatory limitation.

Finally, you should use the blood gas values to calculate the dead-space fraction (V_D/V_T) at each point at which you drew blood gases. This calculation can be done using the following equation:

$$\frac{V_D}{V_T} = \frac{PaCO_2 - P_ECO_2}{PaCO_2}.$$

P_ECO_2 is the mean expired PCO_2 at the time the blood gas was obtained and is usually calculated by the exercise system. It is not the same value as the end-tidal carbon dioxide. The dead-space calculation is important as it provides clues to the presence of a pulmonary vascular/interstitial lung disease pattern of limitation. In normals and in patients with cardiac limitation, V_D/V_T will decrease with exercise to less than 30% while in pulmonary vascular and interstitial lung disease patients, it will remain stable or increase.

PATTERN OF EXERCISE LIMITATION

In this section—which serves as the meat of your test interpretation—you should identify what you believe to be the primary source of the patient's exercise limitation—cardiac problems, ventilatory problems, pulmonary vascular disease, interstitial lung disease, or another process. The different patterns of limitation are described more thoroughly in Chap. 3 and are summarized in Table 5.2. Some texts recommend using a flowchart approach to identify the source of exercise limitation. At our institution, we prefer to use a different approach that is based more on pattern recognition rather than strict decision algorithms.

In some patients, the data from the cardiopulmonary exercise test will be entirely consistent with a particular pattern of limitation and identifying the limiting system is relatively straightforward. In other cases, however, all of the data may not conform entirely to one of the common patterns. For example, a patient may have many elements of cardiac limitation such as a ventilatory threshold, a fall in their $PetCO_2$ at end-exercise, leg fatigue as their primary symptom, and a decrease in their dead-space fraction but their minute ventilation rises very close to or above their predicted maximum ventilation (i.e., a small ventilatory reserve). In such cases, we determine the system that is limiting exercise by seeing where the preponderance of the evidence lies. In the example noted above, because most of the data is consistent with a cardiac limitation pattern and only a single variable, the ventilatory reserve, changes in a manner seen in the ventilatory limitation pattern, we would say that this patient demonstrates cardiac limitation. This concept is illustrated in Fig. 5.6.

When applying this approach, which we refer to as the "balance approach," it is important to note that different weight is attached to each of the variables under consideration. This is demonstrated in Fig. 5.6 by the fact that the boxes are of different sizes. For example, the presence of a ventilatory threshold is a critical variable in identifying the cardiac pattern of limitation and you would be wary of labeling a patient as having ventilatory limitation if there was evidence of a clear threshold. Other variables such as the heart rate reserve carry less weight and are best viewed as being smaller boxes in this approach. With regard to the ventilatory limitation pattern, critical features include a rising $PetCO_2$ at end-exercise and the absence of a

TABLE 5.2 BASIC PATTERNS OF EXERCISE LIMITATION ON CARDIOPULMONARY EXERCISE TESTING

	Patterns of limitation		
Variable	Cardiac[a]	Pulmonary vascular disease/ILD[b]	Ventilatory
Blood pressure	Should rise throughout[c]	Rises throughout	Rises throughout
Dead space (V_D/V_T)[d]	Decreases	Remains stable or increases	Variable decrease[e]
Heart rate reserve	Variable	Small to absent	Large
Metabolic acidosis (late exercise)	Present	Present	Absent
O_2 pulse	May plateau near end-exercise	May plateau near end-exercise	Increases throughout[f]
Oxygen saturation	Stable	May decrease	May decrease
$P_{ET}CO_2$ (late exercise)	Decreased	Decreased	Increased or stable
Reason for stopping	Leg fatigue	Dyspnea, leg fatigue	Dyspnea
Respiratory exchange ratio	Usually exceeds 1.1	Usually exceeds 1.1	Often remains below 1.0
$\dot{V}_E/\dot{V}CO_2$	May be increased[g]	Increased[h]	Increased[i]
Ventilatory reserve	Large	Small	Small–absent
Ventilatory threshold	Present	Present	Absent
$\dot{V}O_{2\,max}$	Decreased[j]	Decreased	Decreased

Variables have been listed in alphabetical order rather than according to the importance in determining the cause of exercise limitation

[a] The normal individual will demonstrate a "cardiac pattern" of limitation. The key factor that distinguishes them from someone with underlying cardiac disease is the fact that the $\dot{V}O_{2\,max}$ will be in the normal range whereas it will be decreased in an individual with underlying cardiac disease

[b] Interstitial lung disease patients demonstrate a pattern very similar to the pulmonary vascular pattern and can only be differentiated based on their PFTs and chest imaging

[c] In some patients with underlying cardiac disease, blood pressure may not rise or may even decrease with progressive exercise, a concerning finding indicative of severe disease

[d] As measured by arterial blood gases. This yields a different and more diagnostically useful value than that reported by many exercise systems that use the end-tidal CO_2 instead of arterial CO_2 in the calculation

[e] V_D/V_T may not decrease in patients who develop severe air-trapping during exercise

[f] Patients with ventilatory limitation may have a plateau in their O_2 pulse if they have severe air-trapping

[g] Increased ventilatory equivalents noted before the ventilatory threshold are suggestive of severe heart failure

[h] This is suggestive of increased dead space

[i] Seen with severe chronic obstructive pulmonary disease with carbon dioxide retention

[j] Normal individuals also demonstrate a cardiac pattern of limitation. The $\dot{V}O_{2\,max}$ in these individuals will be in the normal range as predicted by their age, gender, and height

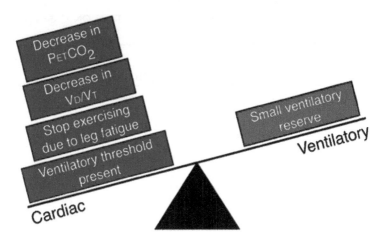

Fig. 5.6 The balance approach to identifying the pattern of exercise limitation. In this example, the patient has many features that are consistent with a cardiac pattern of limitation and only one aspect of their data—the small ventilatory reserve—that is consistent with a ventilatory limitation. Because the preponderance of factors favor the *left side* of the balance, this patient would be best described as having a cardiac pattern or limitation

ventilatory threshold. These would be considered the largest blocks in the balance approach as it applies to this pattern. For the pulmonary vascular disease/interstitial lung disease pattern, the largest block in this balance approach would be failure of the dead-space fraction to decrease through exercise.

FINAL IMPRESSION AND SUMMARY

The discussion of the pattern of exercise limitation can be in its own free-standing section of the report or can go into the final section of the report which we usually title "Impression/Summary." In this section, you will reiterate the main findings of the study, including the maximum oxygen consumption and other key data, and enumerate the reasons why the test subject was felt to demonstrate that particular pattern of exercise limitation.

In this last section of the report, you should also address any specific questions the requesting provider may have had about the individual's exercise performance. For example, if the requesting pro-

TABLE 5.3 SAMPLE SUMMARY DATA TABLE

Measurement	Rest	Max exercise	Predicted max	% Predicted
Work (W)	0	118	129	91%
$\dot{V}O_2$ (ml/min)	242	1,458	1,620	90%
$\dot{V}O_2$/kg (ml/kg/min)	3.0	17.8	19.8	90%
Heart rate (bpm)	81	153	169	91%
O_2 pulse (ml O_2/beat)	3	10	10	99%
Blood pressure (mmHg)	98/60	162/90		
Ventilation (l/min)	8.4	65.9	116	50% of MVV
				57% of $FEV_1 \times 40$
Respiratory rate (bpm)	9	31		
Tidal volume (l)	0.88	2.11		
O_2 saturation (%)	100	100		
$P_{ET}CO_2$ (mmHg)	35	35*		

*$P_{ET}CO_2$ reached 44 at the ventilatory threshold before falling to 35 at the end of the study

vider is trying to determine whether a patient is limited by their underlying heart disease or underlying lung diseases as part of their decision as to whether to proceed with cardiac surgery, you would comment on that issue here. Similarly, if a cardiomyopathy patient was having serial tests over time to follow their exercise capacity in order to facilitate decisions about when to list the patient for heart transplantation, you would include comments about the change in their maximum exercise capacity relative to their prior studies.

SUMMARY DATA TABLE

In addition to the text description that you will include in your report, it is useful to include a data table that summarizes the main results of the study in numerical format. This helps the reader of the report to identify important pieces of information. At our institution, the data table includes the resting values for each parameter, the values seen at peak exercise, the predicted maximum values for that patient, and the percentage of each of the predicted values obtained by the patient. An example of such a summary data table is provided in Table 5.3 and in the sample report in the Appendix to this chapter.

APPENDIX: SAMPLE CARDIOPULMONARY EXERCISE TEST REPORT

CARDIOPULMONARY STRESS TEST INTERPRETATION
Date of Study: 9/21/10

Referring Provider:

Test Performed By:

Indications for Testing: 50-year-old woman with dyspnea on exertion of unclear etiology

Diagnoses:
Dyspnea on exertion
Cough

| Age: 50 | Height: 165 cm | Weight: 81.7 kg | BMI: 30 |

PULMONARY FUNCTION TESTING
Spirometry: FEV_1 2.91 l (105% predicted), FVC 3.44 l (101% predicted), FEV_1/FVC 0.85

Post-bronchodilator Spirometry: Not performed

Maximum Voluntary Ventilation: 131 l/minute

Postexercise spirometry: The FEV_1 remained between 2.77 and 2.91 l at testing performed every 3 minute postexercise up until 20 minute had elapsed. The contour of the inspiratory limb of the flow volume loops during the postexercise testing was irregular but did not show evidence of flattening consistent with an upper airway obstruction.

Interpretation: Normal spirometry. No evidence of airflow obstruction following exercise.

PULMONARY STRESS TEST, COMPLEX
Exercise Protocol: The risks and benefits of progressive maximal cardiopulmonary exercise testing and arterial line placement were explained to the patient. After obtaining consent, an arterial line was placed on the first attempt in the left wrist in a sterile manner using a

modified Seldinger technique. Upon placement of the catheter, the patient was placed on the exercise bicycle and was without symptoms. She was exercised on the cycle ergometer to a symptom-limited maximum with progressively increasing workload at 15-W/minute increments. Continuous oxygen saturation, ECG, and expired gas analysis were performed. Serial blood pressures were obtained. Arterial blood gas samples were obtained prior to the start of exercise and every 2 minute during the exercise test. The patient reached a maximum of 118 W and appeared to give a good effort. She was sweating at the end of the test.

Reason For Stopping Exercise: Leg fatigue. The patient did not develop any coughing similar to what she describes when she is having difficulty with exercise at home or at work.

RESULTS
Summary Data

Measurement	Rest	Max exercise	Predicted max	% Predicted
Work (W)	0	118	129	91
$\dot{V}O_2$ (ml/minute)	242	1,458	1,620	90
$\dot{V}O_2$ / kg (ml/kg/minute)	3.0	17.8	19.8	90
Heart rate (bpm)	81	153	169	91
O_2 pulse (ml O_2/beat)	3	10	10	99
Blood pressure (mmHg)	98/60	162/90		
Ventilation (l/minute)	8.4	65.9	116	50% of MVV
				57% of $FEV_1 \times 40$
Respiratory rate (bpm)	9	31		
Tidal volume (l)	0.88	2.11		
O_2 saturation (%)	100	100		
$P_{ET}CO_2$ (mmHg)	35	35[a]		

[a] $P_{ET}CO_2$ reached 44 at the ventilatory threshold before falling to 35 at the end of the study

Maximum oxygen consumption: The patient's $\dot{V}O_{2\,max}$ was 1,458 ml/minute, which represented 90% of her predicted maximum. When normalized for her body weight of 81 kg, her $\dot{V}O_{2\,max}$ was 17.8 ml/kg/minute which was 90% of her predicted maximum. When normalized for her IBW of only 57 kg given her height of 165 cm, her $\dot{V}O_{2\,max}$ was 25.7 ml/kg/minute. She achieved a maximum work rate of 118 W, which was 91% of her predicted maximum.

Cardiac response: The resting ECG showed a sinus rhythm with a normal rate, normal axis, and intervals. No ischemic changes were noted at maximum exercise. Her heart rate was 81 beats per minute at rest and rose to 153 beats per minute at maximum exercise, which was 91% of her age-predicted maximum. The O_2 pulse rose from 3 ml/beat at rest to 10 ml/beat at maximum exercise, which was 99% of her predicted maximum. Blood pressure rose from 98/60 at rest to 162/90 at maximum exercise. A ventilatory threshold was observed at a $\dot{V}O_2$ of roughly 840 ml/minute, which was about 57% of her $\dot{V}O_{2\,max}$.

Ventilatory response: The patient's resting ventilation was 8.4 l/minute and increased to 65.9 l/minute at maximum exercise, representing only 50% of her MVV and 57% of her $FEV_1 \times 40$. The respiratory rate rose from 9 at rest to 31 at maximum exercise while tidal volume increased from 0.88 to 2.11 l over the course of the test. The patient's ventilatory equivalents for CO_2 were elevated in the mid-30 range while sitting at rest and subsequently declined to the upper 20-range midway through exercise before rising again over the last half of the test. The ventilatory equivalents for O_2 were in the low 30s at rest and then declined into the 20s once exercise began before rising again in the later half of the test.

Gas exchange: The patient's oxygen saturation was 98–100% at rest and 96% at maximal exercise. Her arterial blood gas results were as follows:

Time point	pH	PaCO₂	PaO₂	(A−a)ΔO₂	Lactate	VD/VT
Rest	7.42	39	100	9	0.8	0.36
Max exercise	7.42	30	125	3	8.3	0.10

IMPRESSION/SUMMARY
The patient achieved a $\dot{V}O_{2\,max}$, normalized for her actual body weight, of 17.8 ml/kg/minute, which was 90% of her predicted maximum. The pattern on this test was consistent with a cardiac pattern of limitation. At maximum exercise, she had a large ventilatory reserve, there was no evidence of hypoxemia, and a clear ventilatory threshold was present as indicated by a rise in her ventilatory equivalents and end-tidal oxygen, drop in her arterial carbon dioxide at end-exercise, and development of a lactic acidosis. There was no evidence of chronotropic limitation. The patient's dead-space fraction decreased appropriately at maximum exercise making it unlikely that she has a pulmonary

vascular/interstitial lung disease pattern of limitation. She had no evidence of ventilatory limitation, as evidenced by the fact that her ventilation at peak exercise was only 50% of her MVV and her arterial CO_2 fell at end-exercise. Her postexercise spirometry did not show any decrements in FEV_1 or FVC compared to her pre-exercise spirometry and there was no evidence of flattening of the inspiratory limb of the flow volume loops on these maneuvers.

REFERENCES

1. Wasserman K, Hansen JE, Sue DY, Stringer WW, Whipp BJ. Principles of exercise testing and interpretation. 4th ed. Philadelphia, PA: Lippincott, Williams and Wilkins; 2005.
2. Jones NL. Clinical exercise testing. 4th ed. Philadelphia, PA: Saunders; 1997.

Chapter 6
Sample Cases Demonstrating Basic Patterns of Exercise Limitation

Keywords Air-trapping • Carbon dioxide production • Cardiac limitation • Cardiac output • Chronotropic limitation • Dead space fraction • End-tidal carbon dioxide • End-tidal oxygen • Forced expiratory volume in one second • Forced vital capacity • Heart rate reserve • Home oxygen therapy • Interstitial lung disease • Lung volume reduction surgery • Maximum oxygen consumption • Maximum voluntary ventilation • Minute ventilation • Oxygen consumption • Oxygen pulse (O_2 pulse) • Oxygen saturation • Pulmonary function testing • Pulmonary vascular disease • Respiratory exchange ratio • Right heart catheterization • Tidal volume • Ventilatory equivalents for carbon dioxide • Ventilatory equivalents for oxygen • Ventilatory limitation • Ventilatory reserve • Ventilatory threshold • V-Slope method

INTRODUCTION TO THE SAMPLE CASES

In this section of the primer you will find examples of cardiopulmonary exercise tests that demonstrate each of the four most common patterns of results that you may see over the course of your work in the cardiopulmonary exercise testing laboratory. These four patterns include:

- Cardiac limitation pattern in a subject with no underlying cardiopulmonary disease.
- Cardiac limitation pattern in a subject with known cardiomyopathy.

A.M. Luks et al., *Introduction to Cardiopulmonary Exercise Testing*, DOI 10.1007/978-1-4614-6283-5_6, © Springer Science+Business Media New York 2013

- Ventilatory limitation pattern.
- Pulmonary vascular/interstitial lung disease pattern.

These cases are meant to be representative of the typical patterns you will see in patients with these issues but you should be aware that variations on these themes do occur and some cases you will review will not necessarily fit into these patterns. We will not focus on less common patterns of exercise limitation, such as neuromuscular diseases, for which there is more variability in presentation, making delineation of a single pattern difficult.

While we have simplified the approach to consider a single system as limiting exercise, in reality patients can have both cardiac and pulmonary limitations. In these cases, we try to identify the primary system-limiting exercise and ascribe it to the pattern most consistent with that system. For example, if a patient has both aortic stenosis and chronic obstructive pulmonary disease (COPD), he or she might have an exercise pattern consistent with cardiac limitation if the aortic stenosis was the primary problem. Fixing the aortic stenosis, however, may improve exercise capacity, only to have the patient limited by their COPD. Alternately, improving their COPD symptoms may allow them to improve their maximum exercise capacity, but they would still have cardiac limitation due to their aortic stenosis.

The data in these cases have been taken from exercise tests performed in our laboratory. For each case, we present a summary page that includes the indications for the test, pulmonary function test results, and a table of important data from the exercise test. This summary page is followed by a tabular display of raw data and then by the classic 9-box graphical display of key data from the test. The information in the data tables and 9-box graphical display has been reorganized to improve readability but has the general appearance of the data output you will receive when you interpret exercise tests. For the purpose of keeping the cases concise, the tabular display only includes representative samples of the data from the resting, unloaded pedaling and recovery portions of these studies. In an actual test, you will have all the data from these study portions. We also include a tabular presentation of the key findings in each study that help with identification of the primary pattern of limitation. Finally, each sample case concludes with a brief discussion of the test results and the key learning points that aid in data interpretation.

CASE 1: CARDIAC LIMITATION PATTERN IN A SUBJECT WITH NO UNDERLYING CARDIOPULMONARY DISEASE

Case Description: This is a 38-year-old man who is performing a cardiopulmonary exercise test as part of his orientation to clinical cardiopulmonary exercise testing. He is a physically active person who reports no symptoms of exercise limitation.

Height: 180 cm

Weight: 70 kg

Pretest Pulmonary Function Tests:
FEV_1: 4.65 L (105% predicted)
FVC: 5.88 L (108% predicted)
FEV_1/FVC: 0.79
Maximum voluntary ventilation (MVV): 181 L/minute

Summary Data from Test:

Variable	Rest	Max	Predicted max	% Predicted
Work (W)	0	402	283	142
$\dot{V}O_2$ (ml/minute)	378	4,417	3,146	140
$\dot{V}O_2$ / kg (ml/kg/minute)	5.4	62.8	44.9	140
$\dot{V}O_2$ / kg IBW (ml/kg/minute)	5.4	62.8	44.9	140
Heart rate (bpm)	74	184	185	100
O_2 Pulse (ml O_2/beat)	5.1	23.0	17.0	135
Blood pressure (mmHg)	123/72	175/65		
Ventilation (L/minute)	16	190	181	105% of MVV
				102% of $FEV_1 \times 40$
Respiratory rate (bpm)	16	70		
Tidal volume (L)	0.76	2.5		
O_2 Saturation (%)	98	98		
$P_{ET}CO_2$ (mmHg)	34.9	31.7		

IBW: ideal body weight

Reason for Stopping Test: Leg fatigue

Raw Data from Case 1 Exercise Test

Work (W)	$\dot{V}O_2$ (L/min)	$\dot{V}CO_2$ (L/min)	$\dot{V}E$ (L/min)	HR (bpm)	R	$\dot{V}E/\dot{V}O_2$	$\dot{V}E/\dot{V}CO_2$	$P_{ET}O_2$ (mmHg)	$P_{ET}CO_2$ (mmHg)
Rest	0.38	0.38	16	74	1.01	36	40	111.9	34.9
Unloaded	0.89	0.97	28	90	0.90	35	34	111.2	35.7
5	0.83	0.83	30	93	1.00	35	35	110.0	36.5
15	0.91	0.89	30	88	0.98	32	33	109.1	36.8
21	0.89	0.85	30	89	0.95	32	34	111.8	33.6
30	1.10	1.05	35	92	0.95	31	33	108.8	36.2
35	1.04	1.03	35	96	0.99	33	33	110.9	35.4
45	1.27	1.21	39	98	0.96	30	32	108.2	36.7
55	0.94	0.92	32	101	0.98	33	34	110.4	35.5
61	1.16	1.06	35	100	0.91	30	33	106.2	37.4
70	1.20	1.09	33	98	0.91	27	29	107.2	36.2
80	1.34	1.21	39	104	0.91	28	31	105.6	37.6
85	1.67	1.53	42	109	0.92	29	32	106.0	37.2
95	1.18	1.07	42	113	0.91	29	31	105.8	37.6
105	1.61	1.42	44	119	0.88	27	30	103.6	37.9
110	1.75	1.58	52	120	0.90	29	32	106.4	37.0
120	1.74	1.68	53	126	0.96	30	31	107.5	37.5
125	1.80	1.75	54	131	0.98	30	30	107.9	37.7
136	1.85	1.83	61	131	0.99	32	33	109.5	36.9
146	1.78	1.73	53	127	0.97	29	30	106.6	38.9
150	1.89	1.88	59	126	0.99	31	31	109.1	37.3
160	1.93	1.85	54	127	0.96	28	29	105.0	39.7
171	2.06	1.96	60	134	0.95	29	30	106.1	38.6
176	2.13	2.10	64	132	0.98	29	30	106.9	38.5
186	2.24	2.18	66	138	0.97	29	30	106.9	38.6
190	2.02	1.99	59	142	0.98	29	29	106.1	39.4
201	2.71	2.59	81	148	0.95	30	31	108.5	37.7
211	2.51	2.54	82	147	1.01	32	32	110.7	37.2
216	2.66	2.66	85	148	1.00	31	31	110.5	37.3
226	2.69	2.68	85	150	1.00	31	31	110.2	37.5
231	2.65	2.66	81	148	1.00	30	30	108.8	38.5
241	2.91	2.89	89	151	0.99	30	30	109.6	38.0
246	2.94	2.97	94	158	1.01	31	31	110.8	37.6
256	3.07	3.10	96	160	1.01	31	30	111.2	37.5
266	3.13	3.16	95	161	1.01	30	30	110.4	38.2
271	3.18	3.31	103	163	1.04	32	31	112.3	37.2
286	3.17	3.33	106	163	1.05	33	31	112.7	37.0
291	3.26	3.46	115	165	1.06	35	33	113.9	36.2
296	3.30	3.46	114	165	1.05	34	32	113.2	36.6
311	3.50	3.70	119	167	1.06	34	32	113.6	36.5
311	3.55	3.81	125	169	1.07	35	32	115.0	35.7
321	3.67	3.95	131	169	1.07	35	33	115.4	35.7
326	3.60	4.00	134	171	1.11	37	33	116.1	35.2
336	3.83	4.31	146	175	1.13	38	33	117.1	34.9
346	3.96	4.41	145	177	1.11	36	33	117.0	34.8
353	3.93	4.41	148	175	1.12	37	33	117.4	34.5
361	4.11	4.80	171	180	1.17	41	35	120.1	32.7
369	4.05	4.74	168	182	1.17	41	35	119.8	33.0
377	4.19	4.91	178	184	1.17	42	36	120.7	32.4
385	4.19	4.88	174	182	1.16	41	35	119.8	33.1
393	4.23	4.98	182	184	1.18	43	36	120.7	32.3
402	4.30	5.14	190	184	1.19	44	37	121.5	31.7
1-minute Recovery	1.78	2.77	120	135	1.56	66	43	129.9	27.9
5-minute Recovery	1.06	1.20	61	106	1.14	56	49	125.6	25.4

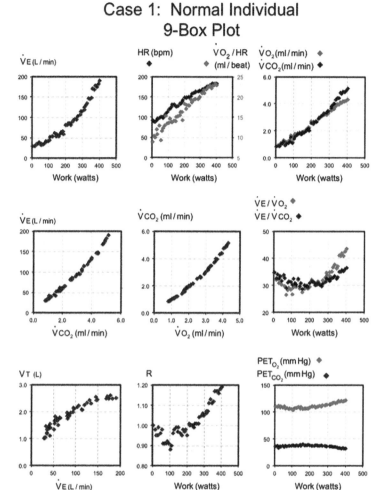

Fig. 6.1 Case 1: Normal individual 9-box plot

TEST INTERPRETATION

The subject exercised to a work rate of 402 W, well above his predicted maximum of 283 W, and achieved a $\dot{V}O_{2\,max}$ of 62.8 ml/kg/minute, which corresponds to 140% of his predicted maximum.

The data demonstrate a cardiac pattern of limitation, the pattern one expects to see in normal individuals with no underlying cardiopulmonary disease. There is a clear ventilatory threshold as demonstrated by the change in the slope of the relationship between $\dot{V}CO_2$ and $\dot{V}O_2$ (V-slope method) and the relationship between $\dot{V}E$ and $\dot{V}CO_2$, the rise in ventilatory equivalents for oxygen ($\dot{V}E/\dot{V}O_2$) and carbon dioxide ($\dot{V}E/\dot{V}CO_2$) in late exercise, and the fact that end-tidal carbon dioxide ($P_{ET}CO_2$) falls in late exercise. The threshold appears to occur around 250–270 W, corresponding to a $\dot{V}O_2$ of about 3.1 L/minute. There is also an appropriate increase in the respiratory exchange ratio and the subject's heart rate at peak exercise was very close to that predicted for him based on his age. Remember that even though this is referred to as a small heart rate reserve, his heart rate at end-exercise is at its maximum and he does not have any "reserve capacity" to raise it further.

At first glance, one might look at the fact that the subject increased his minute ventilation to 105% of his MVV and 102% of his $FEV_1 \times 40$ and think that this small ventilatory reserve was evidence of ventilatory limitation as well. This would not be the correct interpretation with this subject. Fit subjects will often raise their minute ventilation to values near or even above their MVV and appear to have no ventilatory reserve. The key issue for determining if the person actually has ventilatory limitation is what happens with the arterial PCO_2. Because we usually do not have arterial blood gas samples, we use the $P_{ET}CO_2$ as a surrogate for arterial values. In this case, although the subject raises his minute ventilation to just below his MVV, the $P_{ET}CO_2$ decreases progressively as he approaches a maximal effort. In patients with true ventilatory limitation, $P_{ET}CO_2$ will not drop and frequently will rise with maximal effort, in essence demonstrating acute ventilatory failure. You would also not expect to see a clear ventilatory threshold as you do in this case.

Another feature of the data that is worth noting is that the subject has a lower than normal $P_{ET}CO_2$ and somewhat high $\dot{V}E/\dot{V}O_2$ and $\dot{V}E/\dot{V}CO_2$ at rest and with unloaded pedaling. This can sometimes be seen with fit individuals at the start of a cardiopulmonary exercise test, as they are often "amped up" and ready to exercise. This can lead them to hyperventilate to some extent. A similar issue is often seen with nervous individuals. Notice that as he starts exercising the $P_{ET}CO_2$ and ventilatory equivalents return to more normal values as the subject resumes a more appropriate level of minute ventilation. If the high $\dot{V}E/\dot{V}O_2$ and $\dot{V}E/\dot{V}CO_2$ at rest and during unloaded pedaling were due to a pathologic state, such as high dead-space due to pulmonary hypertension, those values would remain high throughout the exercise test.

Table 6.1 outlines the primary findings on the cardiopulmonary exercise test for this patient. You will see that the majority of check marks are found in boxes that correspond to the cardiac pattern of

TABLE 6.1 IDENTIFYING THE PRIMARY PATTERN OF LIMITATION

Observation	This patient	Cardiac	Pulmonary vascular/ILD	Ventilatory
Clear ventilatory threshold	✓	•	•	
Plateau in O_2 pulse (end-exercise)		•	•	•[a]
High $\dot{V}E/\dot{V}CO_2$ (mid-exercise)		•[b]	•	
High $\dot{V}E/\dot{V}O_2$ (mid-exercise)		•[b]	•	
Large ventilatory reserve		•		
Metabolic acidosis by ABG (late exercise)		•	•	
Decreasing $PETCO_2$ (late exercise)	✓	•	•	
R clearly rises above 1.0	✓	•	•	
Stop exercising due to leg fatigue	✓	•	•	
Heart rate near predicted maximum (late exercise)	✓	•[c]		
ST changes on electrocardiography		•		
Inappropriate blood pressure response		•		
Increasing or unchanged V_D/V_T by ABG (late exercise)			•	
Absent ventilatory threshold				•
Decrease in oxygen saturation			•	•
Heart rate far below predicted maximum (late exercise)				•
Increasing or unchanged $PETCO_2$ (late exercise)				•
$PaCO_2$ ≥40 mmHg by ABG (end-exercise)				•
Small ventilatory reserve	✓			•
Decreasing tidal volume				•
R does not increase above 1.0				•
Stop exercising due to dyspnea			•	✓

[a]Can be seen when patients have severe air-trapping leading to increased intrathoracic pressure and decreased venous return

[b]High mid-exercise ventilatory equivalents for carbon dioxide and oxygen can be seen in severe cardiomyopathy. Many patients with cardiac limitation—including normal individuals and those with underlying cardiac disease—may still have normal ventilatory equivalents

[c]Not a reliable observation if the patient is on beta-blockers or has chronotropic limitation

limitation, as would be expected in a normal individual. The one check mark that does not correspond to this pattern is that next to the "small ventilatory reserve box," which, as noted above, can be seen in fit individuals at peak exercise.

CASE 2: CARDIAC LIMITATION PATTERN IN A PATIENT WITH KNOWN CARDIOMYOPATHY

Case Description: This is a 60-year-old woman with known ischemic cardiomyopathy who is undergoing cardiopulmonary exercise testing to follow the progression of her disease and guide decisions regarding when to pursue heart transplantation. She has baseline NYHA Class II symptoms and reports being able to walk one mile on a treadmill in 30 minute. She becomes short of breath climbing one flight of stairs. Her medication regimen includes carvedilol, lisinopril, felodipine, digoxin, and furosemide.

Height: 165 cm

Weight: 86.4 kg

Pretest Pulmonary Function Tests:
FEV_1: 2.15 L (79% predicted)
FVC: 2.96 L (83% predicted)
FEV_1/FVC: 0.73
MVV: 106 L/minute

Summary Data from Test:

Variable	Rest	Max	Predicted max	% Predicted
Work (W)	0	80	109	73
$\dot{V}O_2$ (ml/minute)	390	1,166	1,373	85
$\dot{V}O_2$ / kg (ml/kg/minute)	4.7	14.1	21.3	66
$\dot{V}O_2$ / kg IBW (ml/kg/minute)	6	18.1	21.3	85
Heart rate (bpm)	89	128	159	81
O_2 Pulse (ml O_2/beat)	4.4	9.1	8.6	106
Blood pressure (mmHg)	138/72	172/80		
Ventilation (L/minute)	10	56	106	53% of MVV
				65% of $FEV_1 \times 40$
Respiratory rate (bpm)	14	40		
Tidal volume (L)	0.71	1.4		
O_2 Saturation (%)	97	98		
$PETCO_2$ (mmHg)	41	34		

IBW: ideal body weight

Reason for Stopping Test: Leg fatigue

Raw Data from Case 2 Exercise Test

Work (W)	$\dot{V}O_2$ (L/min)	$\dot{V}CO_2$ (L/min)	$\dot{V}E$ (L/min)	HR (bpm)	R	$\dot{V}E/\dot{V}O_2$	$\dot{V}E/$ $\dot{V}CO_2$	$PETO_2$ (mmHg)	$PETCO_2$ (mmHg)
Rest	0.39	0.31	8	89	0.80	20	25	96	41
Unloaded	0.44	0.47	11	93	0.81	23	27	99	41
0	0.71	0.56	18	94	0.84	25	29	97	41
5	0.38	0.30	18	91	0.80	22	28	98	42
6	0.70	0.61	19	95	0.88	26	30	105	37
11	0.54	0.45	13	92	0.84	23	27	99	41
15	0.63	0.59	18	97	0.92	27	29	105	39
21	0.62	0.59	18	96	0.94	28	30	105	39
21	0.61	0.56	16	96	0.92	26	28	103	40
25	0.65	0.58	17	98	0.89	26	29	101	40
30	0.77	0.70	21	100	0.92	27	29	103	39
30	0.76	0.73	22	100	0.96	28	29	104	39
30	0.75	0.73	21	102	0.96	27	28	104	40
35	0.84	0.83	24	103	0.98	28	29	104	40
40	0.80	0.80	23	105	1.01	28	28	104	40
45	0.84	0.88	27	105	1.05	32	30	107	38
45	0.82	0.85	24	107	1.04	29	28	104	41
50	0.96	1.03	30	109	1.07	31	29	107	39
55	0.92	1.07	33	112	1.16	35	30	109	39
55	0.97	1.12	33	112	1.16	34	29	108	40
55	0.98	1.17	34	113	1.19	34	29	109	40
65	1.00	1.24	38	116	1.24	37	30	112	38
65	1.02	1.29	39	118	1.27	38	31	112	38
70	1.06	1.35	43	120	1.27	39	31	113	38
75	1.07	1.37	43	123	1.29	40	32	114	37
75	1.14	1.50	48	125	1.31	42	34	116	37
80	1.17	1.61	56	128	1.38	47	30	119	34
1 minute Recovery	0.87	1.12	37	109	1.46	48	34	118	36
5 minute Recovery	0.44	0.56	20	99	1.29	44	34	120	32

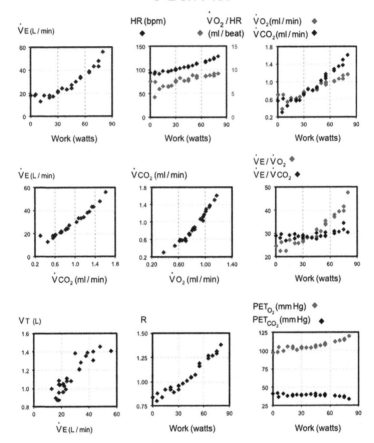

Fig. 6.2 Case 2: Cardiac limitation 9-box plot

TEST INTERPRETATION

This patient demonstrates evidence of mild to moderately reduced exercise capacity. When adjusted for her actual body weight, her $\dot{V}O_{2\,max}$ of 14.1 ml/kg/minute represents 66% of predicted maximum. When normalized for her ideal body weight, her $\dot{V}O_{2\,max}$ of 18.1 ml/kg/minute represents 85% of her predicted maximum.

The data from the test indicate that she has a cardiac pattern as the source of her exercise limitation, a result you would expect given that she has known cardiomyopathy. She demonstrates a ventilatory threshold as evidenced by several factors including the change in the slope of the relationship between $\dot{V}CO_2$ and $\dot{V}O_2$ (i.e., a change in her V-slope), the drop in her $P_{ET}CO_2$ and rise in $P_{ET}O_2$ in late exercise, the marked rise in her respiratory exchange ratio, and the increases in $\dot{V}E / \dot{V}O_2$ and $\dot{V}E/\dot{V}CO_2$ in late exercise. The ventilatory threshold likely occurs around 45 W or a $\dot{V}O_2$ of 0.82 L. The fact that she stopped due to leg fatigue and the absence of oxygen desaturation in late exercise are also consistent with a cardiac source of exercise limitation. The fact that this patient has a cardiac pattern of limitation can be appreciated in Table 6.2, in which all of her check marks fall in boxes corresponding to this pattern.

It is worth noting that the patient's heart rate rose to only 128 beats per minute compared to her age-predicted maximum of 159 beats per minute. Patients with most myocardial diseases will have a reduced chronotropic response compared to healthy age-comparable normal subjects, and this chronotropic abnormality is augmented by treatment with beta blockers.

For this reason, if you perform a cardiopulmonary exercise test on a patient using beta-blockers, the presence of a large difference between their heart rate at peak exercise and the predicted maximum heart rate should not push one away from labeling the patient as having a cardiac pattern of limitation if the other data are consistent with such a pattern. This is one of the reasons why when considering the possibility of cardiac limitation, the heart rate reserve is given less weight in our pattern recognition approach than other variables such as the presence of a ventilatory threshold.

The patient demonstrates no evidence of ventilatory limitation as her minute ventilation at peak exercise is far below her MVV and $FEV_1 \times 40$; she does not experience a fall in her oxygen saturation and, as noted above, there is a fall in her $P_{ET}CO_2$ in late exercise.

TABLE 6.2 IDENTIFYING THE PRIMARY PATTERN OF LIMITATION

Observation	This patient	Cardiac	Pulmonary vascular/ILD	Ventilatory
Clear ventilatory threshold	✓	•	•	
Plateau in O_2 pulse (end-exercise)	✓	•	•	•[a]
High $\dot{V}E/\dot{V}CO_2$ (mid-exercise)		•[b]	•	
High $\dot{V}E/\dot{V}O_2$ (mid-exercise)		•[b]	•	
Large ventilatory reserve	✓	•		
Metabolic acidosis by ABG (late exercise)		•	•	
Decreasing $P\text{ET}CO_2$ (late exercise)	✓	•	•	
R clearly rises above 1.0	✓	•	•	
Stop exercising due to leg fatigue	✓	•	•	
Heart rate near predicted maximum (late exercise)	✓	•[c]		
ST changes on electrocardiography		•		
Inappropriate blood pressure response		•		
Increasing or unchanged $V\text{D}/V\text{T}$ by ABG (late exercise)			•	
Absent ventilatory threshold				•
Decrease in oxygen saturation			•	•
Heart rate far below predicted maximum (late exercise)				•
Increasing or unchanged $P\text{ET}CO_2$ (late exercise)				•
$PaCO_2 \geq 40$ mmHg by ABG (end-exercise)				•
Small ventilatory reserve				•
Decreasing tidal volume				•
R does not increase above 1.0				•
Stop exercising due to dyspnea			•	•

[a]Can be seen when patients have severe air-trapping leading to increased intrathoracic pressure and decreased venous return

[b]High mid-exercise ventilatory equivalents for carbon dioxide and oxygen can be seen in severe cardiomyopathy. Many patients with cardiac limitation—including normal individuals and those with underlying cardiac disease—may still have normal ventilatory equivalents

[c]Not a reliable observation if the patient is on beta-blockers or has chronotropic limitation

CASE 3: VENTILATORY LIMITATION PATTERN

Case Description: This is a 61-year-old man with a history of COPD, who is status-post lung volume reduction surgery and who underwent cardiopulmonary exercise testing as part of the National Emphysema Treatment Trial (NETT). His medications at the time of the test included albuterol and ipratropium metered-dose inhalers and dilti-azem. He was on home oxygen therapy on a continuous basis at a rate of 3 L/minute. The subject was on supplemental oxygen ($F_{I}O_2 = 0.3$) during the test.

Height: 172 cm

Weight: 79 kg

Pretest Pulmonary Function Tests:
FEV_1: 0.43 L (12% predicted)
FVC: 1.91 L (43% predicted)
FEV_1/FVC: 0.23
MVV: 16 L/minute

Summary Data from Test:

Variable	Rest	Max	Predicted max	% Predicted
Work (W)	0	27	158	17
$\dot{V}O_2$ (ml/minute)	339	693	2,120	33
$\dot{V}O_2$ / kg (ml/kg/minute)	4.3	8.1	31.3	26
$\dot{V}O_2$ / kg IBW (ml/kg/minute)	5.1	10.3	31.6	32
Heart rate (bpm)	82	111	158	70
O_2 Pulse (ml O_2/beat)	4	5.8	13	44
Blood pressure (mmHg)	150/90	180/110		
Ventilation (L/minute)	10	16	16	100% of MVV
				93% of $FEV_1 \times 40$
Respiratory rate (bpm)	17	34		
Tidal volume (L)	0.87	0.77		
O_2 Saturation (%)	98%	93%		
$P_{ET}CO_2$ (mmHg)	45	57		

IBW: ideal body weight

Reason for Stopping Test: Dyspnea

Raw Data from Case 3 Exercise Test

Work (W)	$\dot{V}O_2$ (L/min)	$\dot{V}CO_2$ (L/min)	$\dot{V}_E$ (L/min)	HR (bpm)	R	$\dot{V}_E/\dot{V}O_2$	$\dot{V}_E/\dot{V}CO_2$	PETO$_2$ (mmHg)	PETCO$_2$ (mmHg)
Rest	0.34	0.27	10	82	0.80	31	38	164	45
Unloaded	0.41	0.32	13	94	0.72	28	39	152	48
1	0.51	0.37	14	96	0.73	27	38	151	50
2	0.51	0.37	14	96	0.73	27	37	152	50
5	0.52	0.37	13	94	0.72	25	35	149	52
6	0.50	0.36	13	97	0.73	27	37	150	51
8	0.52	0.38	14	100	0.73	27	37	150	51
9	0.56	0.40	14	99	0.72	25	35	149	52
11	0.57	0.41	14	99	0.72	24	34	148	52
13	0.56	0.41	14	99	0.73	26	35	150	52
15	0.56	0.41	15	98	0.73	26	36	149	52
16	0.56	0.40	14	99	0.71	25	35	148	52
19	0.58	0.42	15	102	0.73	26	36	150	53
20	0.61	0.44	15	103	0.72	24	34	146	53
21	0.62	0.45	15	102	0.72	24	34	148	54
23	0.64	0.46	15	106	0.72	23	32	146	54
25	0.64	0.46	16	107	0.73	25	34	147	55
27	0.64	0.47	16	111	0.72	25	34	146	57
1-minute Recovery	0.68	0.49	15	105	0.73	22	30	142	57
3-minute Recovery	0.56	0.44	14	100	0.79	26	33	149	55

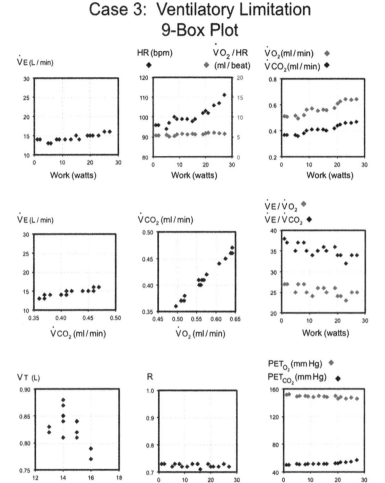

Fig. 6.3 Case 3: Ventilatory limitation 9-box plot

TEST INTERPRETATION

This patient has a markedly reduced maximum exercise capacity. When normalized for his actual body weight, his $\dot{V}O_{2\,max}$ of 8.1 ml/kg/ minute represents only 26% of his predicted maximum and when normalized for his ideal body weight, his $\dot{V}O_{2\,max}$ of 10.3 ml/kg/minute represents only 32% of his predicted maximum. This represents a significant degree of impairment.

The data in this case are consistent with a ventilatory pattern of exercise limitation. The patient's minute ventilation at peak exercise is 100% of his MVV and 93% of his $FEV_1 \times 40$. This indicates that he has no ventilatory reserve at end-exercise. In addition, rather than decreasing in the later stages of exercise, as happens in people with cardiac or pulmonary vascular/interstitial lung disease patterns of limitation, his $P_{ET}CO_2$ rises throughout exercise. In fact, his $P_{ET}CO_2$ was elevated at rest and began rising relative to resting values during unloaded pedaling, indicating that he was already experiencing a mild degree of ventilatory failure during this stage of the test. It is also noteworthy that his tidal volumes fell between the start and end of loaded pedaling, a fact that suggests that he is developing progressive air-trapping and/or respiratory muscle fatigue over the course of the test. Air-trapping is a phenomenon that can develop during exercise in patients with severe obstructive lung disease as the increasing respiratory rate during exercise shortens exhalation time and prevents complete emptying of the lungs. Despite using supplemental oxygen, the patient also experiences a drop in his oxygen saturation during the test, a finding, which can be seen in patients with either ventilatory or pulmonary vascular/interstitial lung disease patterns of exercise limitation. The consistency of the data with a ventilatory limitation pattern can be appreciated in Table 6.3.

There is no evidence in this test that would fit with a cardiac pattern of limitation. He has no definable ventilatory threshold. Notice that his minute ventilation does not increase in late exercise, nor is there a change in the slope of the $\dot{V}CO_2$ vs. $\dot{V}O_2$ or $\dot{V}E$ vs. $\dot{V}CO_2$ relationships that is typically seen when the ventilatory threshold is reached. This occurs because he is unable to raise his minute ventilation due to his severely impaired respiratory mechanics. His respiratory exchange ratio, $\dot{V}E / \dot{V}O_2$ and $\dot{V}E/\dot{V}CO_2$, also do not increase in late exercise. In fact, the ventilatory equivalent values fall towards the end of the test as he goes into overt ventilatory failure; minute ventilation cannot be increased to match the rise in carbon dioxide production and oxygen consumption. Finally, he has a large heart rate reserve at end-exercise, as his heart rate reached only 70% of his age-predicted maximum. This supports the conclusion that he can no longer exercise because his respiratory system has failed long before his heart would have limited his ability to exercise.

TABLE 6.3 IDENTIFYING THE PRIMARY PATTERN OF LIMITATION

Observation	This patient	Cardiac	Pulmonary vascular/ILD	Ventilatory
			Pattern of limitation	
Clear ventilatory threshold		•	•	
Plateau in O_2 pulse (end exercise)		•	•	•[a]
High $\dot{V}E/\dot{V}CO_2$ (mid-exercise)		•[b]	•	
High $\dot{V}E/\dot{V}O_2$ (mid-exercise)		•[b]	•	
Large ventilatory reserve		•		
Metabolic acidosis by ABG (late exercise)		•	•	
Decreasing $PETCO_2$ (late exercise)		•	•	
R clearly rises above 1.0		•	•	
Stop exercising due to leg fatigue		•	•	
Heart rate near predicted maximum (late exercise)		•[c]		
ST changes on electrocardiography		•		
Inappropriate blood pressure response		•		
Increasing or unchanged VD/VT by ABG (late exercise)			•	
Absent ventilatory threshold	✓			•
Decrease in oxygen saturation	✓		•	•
Heart rate far below predicted maximum (late exercise)	✓			•
Increasing or unchanged $PETCO_2$ (late exercise)	✓			•
$PaCO \geq 40$ mmHg by ABG (end-exercise)				•
Small ventilatory reserve	✓			•
Decreasing tidal volume	✓			•
R does not increase above 1.0	✓			•
Stop exercising due to dyspnea	✓		•	•

[a]Can be seen when patients have severe air-trapping leading to increased intrathoracic pressure and decreased venous return

[b]High mid-exercise ventilatory equivalents for carbon dioxide and oxygen can be seen in severe cardiomyopathy. Many patients with cardiac limitation—including normal individuals and those with underlying cardiac disease—may still have normal ventilatory equivalents

[c]Not a reliable observation if the patient is on beta-blockers or has chronotropic limitation

CASE 4: PULMONARY VASCULAR/ INTERSTITIAL LUNG DISEASE PATTERN

Case Description: This is a 59-year-old man diagnosed with Sarcoidosis 25 years ago who was referred for cardiopulmonary exercise testing to evaluate dyspnea on exertion and decreasing exercise tolerance over a several month period. His oxygen saturation has been noted to fall with walking on flat ground. His prior workup included an echocardiogram, which revealed evidence of a patent foramen ovale and a right heart catheterization, which showed evidence of mild pulmonary hypertension. He is on home oxygen and also uses CPAP for obstructive sleep apnea. His baseline hematocrit is 53%.

Height: 165 cm

Weight: 131 kg

Pretest Pulmonary Function Tests:
FEV_1: 1.79 L (56% predicted)
FVC: 2.61 L (65% predicted)
FEV_1/FVC: 0.69
MVV: 74 L/minute

Summary Data from Test:

Variable	Rest	Max	Predicted max	% Predicted
Work (W)	0	85	157	54
$\dot{V}O_2$ (ml/minute)	348	1,527	2,597	59
$\dot{V}O_2$ / kg (ml/kg/minute)	2.6	11.6	28.9	40
$\dot{V}O_2$ / kg IBW (ml/kg/minute)	5.6	24.5	28.9	85
Heart rate (bpm)	75	135	161	84
O_2 Pulse (ml O_2/beat)	4.6	11.3	11.2	101
Blood pressure (mmHg)	126/76	157/76		
Ventilation (L/minute)	14	67.8	74	92% of MVV
				95% of $FEV_1 \times 40$
Respiratory rate (bpm)	22	51		
Tidal volume (L)	0.64	1.33		
O_2 Saturation (%)	96	90		
$PETCO_2$ (mmHg)	38	35		
VD/VT	0.41	0.56		

IBW: ideal body weight

Reason for Stopping Test: Leg fatigue

Raw Data from Case 4 Exercise Test

Work (W)	$\dot{V}O_2$ (L/min)	$\dot{V}CO_2$ (L/min)	$\dot{V}E$ (L/min)	HR (bpm)	R	$\dot{V}E/\dot{V}O_2$	$\dot{V}E/\dot{V}CO_2$	$PETO_2$ (mmHg)	$PETCO_2$ (mmHg)
Rest	0.31	0.32	11.5	89	1.06	40	38	109	40
Unloaded	0.96	0.98	29.8	97	1.02	31	31	107	41
8	0.95	1.01	31.4	99	1.06	33	31	109	41
6	0.94	0.98	28.9	98	1.05	31	29	107	42
6	0.93	1.00	30.1	99	1.07	32	30	108	41
10	0.86	0.92	28.5	99	1.07	33	31	110	40
15	0.94	0.99	31.8	99	1.05	34	32	110	40
15	0.94	1.01	31.5	100	1.08	34	31	110	40
20	0.92	0.96	29.8	101	1.05	33	31	108	41
24	0.99	1.04	33.2	102	1.05	34	32	110	40
27	0.97	1.04	32.2	102	1.06	33	31	109	41
30	0.98	1.03	32.4	104	1.06	33	31	109	40
33	1.07	1.10	34.4	106	1.03	32	31	108	41
36	1.09	1.17	35.4	108	1.07	33	30	109	40
40	1.11	1.16	34.7	107	1.04	31	30	108	41
43	1.11	1.18	36.9	108	1.06	33	31	109	41
46	1.16	1.24	39.1	109	1.07	34	32	110	40
50	1.24	1.30	40.6	111	1.05	33	31	109	40
54	1.26	1.37	43.5	113	1.09	35	32	112	39
55	1.30	1.39	45.0	114	1.08	35	32	111	40
60	1.30	1.45	45.8	119	1.11	35	32	112	39
64	1.31	1.46	47.5	123	1.11	36	33	113	38
67	1.33	1.52	48.8	127	1.14	37	32	113	38
70	1.44	1.64	52.9	130	1.14	37	32	114	38
73	1.48	1.70	55.3	135	1.15	37	32	114	38
76	1.47	1.72	57.4	135	1.17	39	34	116	37
80	1.53	1.82	59.5	123	1.19	39	33	117	37
85	1.52	1.88	67.8	120	1.24	45	36	120	35
1 minute Recovery	1.25	1.62	53	129	1.29	42	32	118	37
5 minute Recovery	0.79	1.03	35.6	107	1.30	45	35	118	35

Arterial Blood Gas Data

Time	$PaCO_2$	$PETCO_2$	PaO_2	PAO_2	$(A-a)\Delta O_2$	VD/VT
Unloaded	45	26	74	108	34	0.41
02:20	45	18	72	107	35	0.59
03:20	44	18	68	107	39	0.57
05:00	38	18	67	113	46	0.50
Max exercise	42	18	60	113	53	0.56

Case 4: Limitation Due to Pulmonary Vascular Disease or Interstitial Lung Disease   9-Box Plot

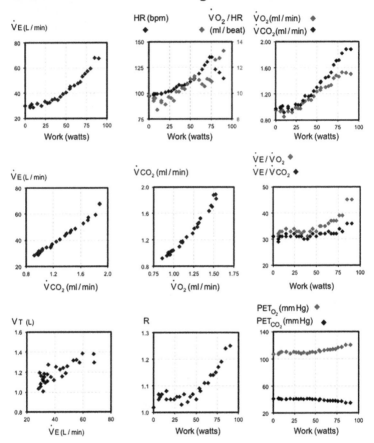

Fig. 6.4 Case 4: Limitation due to pulmonary vascular disease or interstitial lung disease 9-box plot

TEST INTERPRETATION

This patient has evidence of significant exercise limitation. He achieves only 54% of his predicted work rate and, when adjusted for his body weight, his $\dot{V}O_{2\,max}$ is only 40% of his predicted maximum. Even when adjusted for his ideal body weight, his $\dot{V}O_{2\,max}$ represents only 85% of his predicted maximum.

The pattern of data strongly suggests that his exercise limitation is due to pulmonary vascular or interstitial lung disease (ILD). There are several features of this case that are consistent with this finding. He has a ventilatory threshold as evidenced by the rise in his minute ventilation ($\dot{V}E$), $\dot{V}E/\dot{V}CO_2$ and $\dot{V}E/\dot{V}O_2$, as well as the decrease in $PETCO_2$ and rise in $PETO_2$ in late exercise (seen both in the numerical data and on the graphical displays).

While these findings are also seen in patients with cardiac limitation, there are two key findings that distinguish this patient's pattern of results from that of cardiac limitation. First, his oxygen saturation falls during exercise from a baseline of 96 to 90% and his alveolar-arterial oxygen difference widens more than expected. Second, and perhaps most important, his dead-space fraction (VD/VT) increases from 0.41 at rest to 0.56 at peak exercise. In patients with cardiac limitation, oxygen saturation remains constant and VD/VT falls with increasing levels of work. The patient's minute ventilation did rise close to his MVV and $FEV_1 \times 40$ but he managed to decrease his $PaCO_2$ in late exercise, indicating that he was not experiencing ventilatory failure. The minute ventilation requirements are likely increased in this individual due to an elevated dead-space fraction.

The consistency of the data with a pulmonary vascular disease/ILD pattern of limitation can be appreciated in Table 6.4. In general, pulmonary vascular and interstitial lung disease look very similar on cardiopulmonary exercise testing and can only be distinguished from each other with pulmonary function testing and/or a chest CT scan. In this particular case, the fact that he has a prior right heart catheterization showing evidence of pulmonary hypertension points one in the direction of pulmonary vascular disease. In addition, with his obesity, mild baseline hypercarbia ($PaCO_2$ 45 mmHg), and obstructive sleep apnea, one might suspect that he has obesity hypoventilation, which also contributes to elevated pulmonary artery pressures. Sarcoidosis can, however, be associated with ILD, so chest imaging would likely be necessary to determine whether this or pulmonary vascular disease was primarily responsible for his exercise limitation.

TABLE 6.4 IDENTIFYING THE PRIMARY PATTERN OF LIMITATION

Observation	This patient	Cardiac	Pulmonary vascular/ILD	Ventilatory
Clear ventilatory threshold	✓	•	•	
Plateau in O_2 pulse (end exercise)	✓	•	•	•[a]
High $\dot{V}E/\dot{V}CO_2$ (mid-exercise)		•[b]	•	
High $\dot{V}E/\dot{V}O_2$ (mid-exercise)		•[b]	•	
Large ventilatory reserve		•		
Metabolic acidosis by ABG (late exercise)		•	•	
Decreasing $P_{ET}CO_2$ (late exercise)	✓	•	•	
R clearly rises above 1.0	✓	•	•	
Stop exercising due to leg fatigue	✓	•	•	
Heart rate near predicted maximum (late exercise)	✓	•[c]		
ST changes on electrocardiography		•		
Inappropriate blood pressure response		•		
Increasing or unchanged V_D/V_T by ABG (late exercise)	✓		•	
Absent ventilatory threshold				•
Decrease in oxygen saturation	✓		•	•
Heart rate far below predicted maximum (late exercise)				•
Increasing or unchanged $P_{ET}CO_2$ (late exercise)				•
$PaCO_2$ ≥40 mmHg by ABG (end-exercise)				•
Small ventilatory reserve	✓			•
Decreasing tidal volume				•
R does not increase above 1.0				•
Stop exercising due to dyspnea			•	•

[a]Can be seen when patients have severe air-trapping leading to increased intrathoracic pressure and decreased venous return

[b]High mid-exercise ventilatory equivalents for carbon dioxide and oxygen can be seen in severe cardiomyopathy. Many patients with cardiac limitation—including normal individuals and those with underlying cardiac disease—may still have normal ventilatory equivalents

[c]Not a reliable observation if the patient is on beta-blockers or has chronotropic limitation

Chapter 7
Self-Assessment Cases

Keywords Carbon dioxide production • Cardiac limitation • Cardiac output • Chronotropic limitation • Dead space fraction • Echocardiography • End-tidal carbon dioxide • End-tidal oxygen • Eosinophilic granuloma • Forced expiratory volume in one second • Forced vital capacity • Heart rate reserve • Interstitial lung disease • Lung volume reduction surgery • Maximum oxygen consumption • Maximum voluntary ventilation • Minute ventilation • Oxygen consumption • Oxygen pulse (O_2 pulse) • Oxygen saturation • Pulmonary function testing • Pulmonary vascular disease • Respiratory exchange ratio • Right heart catheterization • Sarcoidosis • Tidal volume • Ventilatory equivalents for carbon dioxide • Ventilatory equivalents for oxygen • Ventilatory limitation • Ventilatory reserve • Ventilatory threshold • V-Slope method

INTRODUCTION TO SELF-ASSESSMENT CASES

This last section of the primer is designed to test your skills at cardiopulmonary exercise test interpretation. Five cases are included in this section. The data in each case are presented in a manner similar to the way examples of the various patterns of exercise limitation were presented in the previous chapter, including summary data, raw data from the exercise test itself, and the 9-box plots. Each data set is then followed by a test interpretation worksheet you can use to guide your assessment of the data and determine the primary source of exercise

A.M. Luks et al., *Introduction to Cardiopulmonary Exercise Testing*, DOI 10.1007/978-1-4614-6283-5_7, © Springer Science+Business Media New York 2013

limitation. Explanations regarding the data and the primary pattern of limitation for all of the cases are then provided at the end of this section.

As you interpret the data and try to determine the primary source of exercise limitation, it is important to remember that while each of the basic patterns has classic findings, in many cases, the data from a particular patient will not always conform precisely to these classic or typical findings. For example, the minute ventilation at peak exercise may be close to the maximum voluntary ventilation (>80% of the MVV) even though the patient has cardiac limitation. Situations like this occur relatively frequently in clinical practice.

As a result, when you use the test interpretation worksheet provided with each case to identify the primary pattern of limitation, you will see that your check marks may fall in boxes consistent with different patterns of limitation. As was stressed earlier in the primer in the chapter on test interpretation (Chap. 5) in such cases you should apply the concept of a balance and see where the *preponderance* of evidence lies and use that as the means to determine what the primary pattern of exercise limitation is for a particular case. Check marks may fall in boxes consistent with multiple patterns of limitation but the majority of check marks will reside within boxes corresponding to the primary limiting process. By far the most important box is the presence of a ventilatory threshold.

SELF-ASSESSMENT CASE 1

Case Description: This is a 50-year-old woman who has been referred for cardiopulmonary exercise testing for worsening exercise tolerance. She notes increasing dyspnea on exertion but states that the bigger problem is that right at the end of exercise she becomes very lightheaded and almost passes out. She adds that the symptoms persist for several minutes following exercise and "it is all I can do to keep from falling off the bicycle."

Height: 170 cm

Weight: 76 kg

Pretest Pulmonary Function Tests:
FEV_1: 3.10 L (105% predicted)
FVC: 4.28 L (116% predicted)
FEV_1/FVC: 0.72
Maximum voluntary ventilation: 121 L/minute

Summary Data from Test:

Variable	Rest	Max	Predicted max	% Predicted
Work (W)	0	156	186	83
$\dot{V}O_2$ (ml/minute)	250	1,907	2,297	83
$\dot{V}O_2$ / kg (ml/kg/minute)	3.3	25.3	34.7	73
$\dot{V}O_2$ / kg IBW (ml/kg/minute)	3.8	28.8	34.7	83
Heart rate (bpm)	89	161	170	95
O_2 Pulse (ml O_2/beat)	2.8	11.8	13.5	88
Blood pressure (mmHg)	102/76	122/78		
Ventilation (L/minute)	10	101	121	83% of MVV
				81% of $FEV_1 \times 40$
Respiratory rate (bpm)	12	41		
Tidal volume (L)	0.83	2.46		
O_2 Saturation (%)	100	100		
$P_{ET}CO_2$ (mmHg)	32	28		
V_D/V_T	0.29	0.18		

IBW: ideal body weight

ECG Results: No evidence of ischemia. No arrhythmia.

Reason for Stopping Test: Dyspnea. The patient's pre-syncopal symptoms were recreated at the end of this test and she had to be held up and prevented from falling off the bicycle. Her blood pressure at this time was 90/72.

Raw Data from Case 1 Exercise Test

Work (W)	$\dot{V}O_2$ (L/min)	$\dot{V}CO_2$ (L/min)	$\dot{V}E$ (L/min)	HR (bpm)	R	$\dot{V}E/\dot{V}O_2$	$\dot{V}E/\dot{V}CO_2$	$P_{ET}O_2$ (mmHg)	$P_{ET}CO_2$ (mmHg)
Rest	0.26	0.22	12	94	0.85	31	37	115	32
Unloaded	0.60	0.46	15	98	0.76	24	32	105	34
5	0.56	0.42	13	100	0.74	22	30	101	36
11	0.69	0.51	15	102	0.74	22	30	98	37
15	0.62	0.50	15	98	0.80	24	31	102	36
25	0.58	0.43	13	100	0.75	22	29	100	36
30	0.66	0.48	14	102	0.73	21	29	99	37
35	0.72	0.50	14	105	0.69	19	27	96	38
40	0.91	0.68	20	106	0.75	21	29	98	37
50	0.80	0.59	17	106	0.74	20	27	96	39
55	0.91	0.68	19	109	0.75	21	28	93	40
61	0.99	0.77	21	113	0.78	21	26	96	40
70	0.99	0.78	21	116	0.80	21	26	95	41
75	1.18	0.95	24	120	0.80	20	25	93	42
80	1.15	0.97	25	120	0.84	21	25	96	41
90	1.30	1.10	27	122	0.85	21	25	95	43
95	1.37	1.19	29	125	0.87	21	24	95	44
101	1.43	1.28	30	128	0.89	21	23	94	45
105	1.48	1.35	31	133	0.91	21	23	96	45
116	1.46	1.37	33	136	0.94	22	23	96	46
121	1.58	1.54	35	139	0.97	22	23	96	47
125	1.70	1.73	39	142	1.02	23	22	97	48
130	1.81	1.91	44	145	1.06	24	23	99	47
141	1.87	2.22	59	150	1.19	31	26	110	41
146	1.78	2.37	71	156	1.33	39	30	117	37
156	1.91	2.55	88	153	1.34	46	34	123	31
156	1.88	2.61	101	161	1.39	53	38	126	28
1-minute Recovery	1.05	1.47	54	133	1.41	55	39	125	28
2-minute Recovery	0.81	1.19	47	130	1.47	57	39	125	30

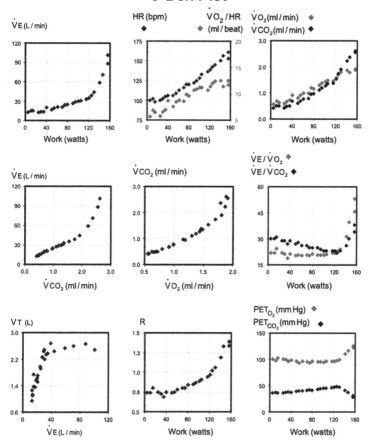

Fig. 7.1 Self-assessment case 1: 9-box plot

SELF-ASSESSMENT CASE 1: EXERCISE TEST INTERPRETATION WORKSHEET

Review the data from the test and provide your best assessment for each of the following variables:

Observation	This patient	Cardiac	Pulmonary vascular/ILD	Ventilatory
Clear ventilatory threshold		•	•	
Plateau in O_2 pulse (end-exercise)		•	•	•[a]
High ($\dot{V}E / \dot{V}CO_2$) (mid-exercise)		•[b]	•	
High ($\dot{V}E / \dot{V}O_2$) (mid-exercise)		•[b]	•	
Large ventilatory reserve		•		
Metabolic acidosis by ABG (late exercise)		•	•	
Decreasing $PETCO_2$ (late exercise)		•	•	
R clearly rises above 1.0		•	•	
Stop exercising due to leg fatigue		•	•	
Heart rate near predicted maximum (late exercise)		•[c]		
ST changes on electrocardiography		•		
Inappropriate blood pressure response		•		
Increasing or unchanged VD/VT by ABG (late exercise)			•	
Absent ventilatory threshold				•
Decrease in oxygen saturation			•	•
Heart rate far below predicted maximum (late exercise)				•
Increasing or unchanged $PETCO_2$ (late exercise)				•
$PaCO_2$ ≥40 mmHg by ABG (end-exercise)				•
Small ventilatory reserve				•
Decreasing tidal volume				•
R does not increase above 1.0				•
Stop exercising due to dyspnea			•	•

[a] Can be seen when patients have severe air-trapping leading to increased intrathoracic pressure and decreased venous return

[b] High mid-exercise ventilatory equivalents for carbon dioxide and oxygen can be seen in severe cardiomyopathy. Many patients with cardiac limitation—including normal individuals and those with underlying cardiac Vdisease—may still have normal ventilatory equivalents

[c] Not a reliable observation if the patient is on beta-blockers or has chronotropic limitation

Describe the $\dot{V}O_{2\,max}$:   Normal (>80% predicted): ____
                          Decreased (<80% predicted): ____

What do you think is the primary pattern of exercise limitation for this patient?

- Cardiac: ____
- Ventilatory: ____
- Pulmonary Vascular/Interstitial Lung Disease: ____

What testing or further evaluation should you pursue to follow up the results of this test?

SELF-ASSESSMENT CASE 2

Case Description: This is a 61-year-old man who was diagnosed with eosinophilic granuloma (Langerhan's cell histiocytosis) several years ago. He has continued to smoke cigarettes since that time and now presents with worsening dyspnea on exertion.

Height: 175 cm

Weight: 82 kg

Pretest Pulmonary Function Tests:
FEV_1: 2.69 L (75% predicted)
FVC: 3.54 L (77% predicted)
FEV_1/FVC: 0.76
Maximum voluntary ventilation: 133 L/minute

Summary Data from Test:

Variable	Rest	Max	Predicted max	% Predicted
Work (W)	0	102	206	49
$\dot{V}O_2$ (ml/minute)	326	1,476	2,700	55
$\dot{V}O_2$ / kg (ml/kg/minute)	4.0	18.1	33.1	55
Heart rate (bpm)	73	138	159	86
O_2 Pulse (ml O_2/beat)	4	11	17	62
Blood pressure (mmHg)	112/82	168/91		
Ventilation (L/minute)	15	72	133	54% of MVV
				66% of $FEV_1 \times 40$
Respiratory rate (bpm)	14	37		
Tidal volume (L)	1.1	2.1		
O_2 Saturation (%)	97	92		
$PETCO_2$ (mmHg)	30	28		
V_D/V_T	0.48	0.43		

ECG Results: No evidence of ischemia. No arrhythmia

Reason for Stopping Test: Leg fatigue, dyspnea

Raw Data from Case 2 Exercise Test

Work (W)	$\dot{V}O_2$ (L/min)	$\dot{V}CO_2$ (L/min)	$\dot{V}E$ (L/min)	HR (bpm)	R	$\dot{V}E/\dot{V}O_2$	$\dot{V}E/\dot{V}CO_2$	$P_{ET}O_2$ (mmHg)	$P_{ET}CO_2$ (mmHg)
Rest	0.33	0.30	16	73	0.93	48	52	112	30
Unloaded	0.56	0.45	19	82	0.80	34	43	106	31
2	0.60	0.57	23	85	0.94	38	41	109	31
8	0.58	0.55	23	87	0.95	40	42	109	31
12	0.60	0.56	23	89	0.93	39	42	108	32
19	0.68	0.65	27	88	0.95	39	41	109	32
21	0.64	0.60	24	90	0.93	37	40	107	33
27	0.64	0.63	26	91	0.97	40	42	110	32
32	0.76	0.71	28	91	0.94	38	40	108	32
39	0.73	0.70	29	93	0.96	39	41	110	31
41	0.76	0.75	30	95	0.98	40	41	110	31
48	0.79	0.75	30	97	0.95	38	40	108	32
52	0.86	0.86	35	99	1.01	41	41	111	30
58	0.91	0.91	37	104	1.00	40	40	110	31
62	0.93	0.97	40	108	1.04	43	42	112	30
67	1.02	1.03	41	111	1.01	40	40	111	31
73	1.09	1.16	47	113	1.06	43	40	113	30
78	1.12	1.19	47	119	1.06	42	40	112	31
82	1.20	1.35	56	122	1.12	47	41	115	29
89	1.28	1.38	55	124	1.07	43	40	115	30
92	1.35	1.51	60	127	1.12	44	40	115	30
98	1.39	1.62	67	134	1.16	48	41	117	29
102	1.45	1.72	72	138	1.19	49	42	118	28
1-minute Recovery	1.27	1.58	65.4	134	1.24	52	41	119	28

Arterial Blood Gas Data

Time	$PaCO_2$	$P_{ET}CO_2$	PaO_2	P_AO_2	$(A-a)\Delta O_2$	Lactate	V_D/V_T
Rest	36	29	89	108	19	0.9	0.48
Max exercise	38	28	71	114	43	7.6	0.43

Self Assessment Case 2
9-Box Plot

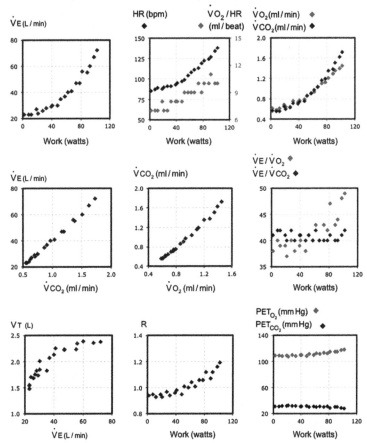

Fig. 7.2 Self-assessment case 2: 9-box plot

SELF-ASSESSMENT CASE 2: EXERCISE TEST INTERPRETATION WORKSHEET

Review the data from the test and provide your best assessment for each of the following variables:

Observation	This patient	Cardiac	Pulmonary vascular/ILD	Ventilatory
			Pattern of limitation	
Clear ventilatory threshold		•	•	
Plateau in O_2 pulse (end-exercise)		•	•	•[a]
High ($\dot{V}E / \dot{V}CO_2$)(mid-exercise)		•[b]	•	
High ($\dot{V}E / \dot{V}O_2$)(mid-exercise)		•[b]	•	
Large ventilatory reserve		•		
Metabolic acidosis by ABG (late exercise)		•	•	
Decreasing $P\text{ET}CO_2$ (late exercise)		•	•	
R clearly rises above 1.0		•	•	
Stop exercising due to leg fatigue		•	•	
Heart rate near predicted maximum (late exercise)		•[c]		
ST changes on electrocardiography		•		
Inappropriate blood pressure response		•		
Increasing or unchanged V_D/V_T by ABG (late exercise)			•	
Absent ventilatory threshold				•
Decrease in oxygen saturation			•	•
Heart rate far below predicted maximum (late exercise)				•
Increasing or unchanged $P\text{ET}CO_2$ (late exercise)				•
$PaCO_2 \geq 40$ mmHg by ABG (end-exercise)				•
Small ventilatory reserve				•
Decreasing tidal volume				•
R does not increase above 1.0				•
Stop exercising due to dyspnea			•	•

[a]Can be seen when patients have severe air-trapping leading to increased intrathoracic pressure and decreased venous return
[b]High mid-exercise ventilatory equivalents for carbon dioxide and oxygen can be seen in severe cardiomyopathy. Many patients with cardiac limitation—including normal individuals and those with underlying cardiac disease—may still have normal ventilatory equivalents
[c]Not a reliable observation if the patient is on beta-blockers or has chronotropic limitation

Describe the $\dot{V}O_{2max}$: Normal (>80% predicted): ____
Decreased (<80% predicted): ____

What do you think is the primary pattern of exercise limitation for this patient?
- Cardiac: ____
- Ventilatory: ____
- Pulmonary Vascular/Interstitial Lung Disease: ____

What testing or further evaluation should you pursue to follow up the results of this test?

SELF-ASSESSMENT CASE 3

Case Description: 75-year-old man who has been referred for cardio-pulmonary exercise testing for evaluation of dyspnea of unclear etiology.

Height: 188 cm

Weight: 95 kg

Pretest Pulmonary Function Tests:
FEV_1: 2.67 L
FVC: 3.98 L
FEV_1/FVC: 0.67
Maximum voluntary ventilation: 85 L/minute

Summary Data from Test:

Variable	Rest	Max	Predicted max	% Predicted
Work (W)	0	101	177	57
$\dot{V}O_2$ (ml/minute)	365	1,635	2,634	62
$\dot{V}O_2$ / kg (ml/kg/minute)	3.8	17.1	32.8	52
$\dot{V}O_2$ / kg IBW (ml/kg/minute)	4.5	20.4	32.8	62
Heart rate (bpm)	79	104	145	72
O_2 Pulse (ml O_2/beat)	4.6	15.7	18.2	87
Blood pressure (mmHg)	95/55	125/70		
Ventilation (L/minute)	15	76	85	89% of MVV
				71% of $FEV_1 \times 40$
Respiratory rate (bpm)	21	40		
Tidal volume (L)	0.71	1.9		
O_2 Saturation (%)	97	95		
$P_{ET}CO_2$ (mmHg)	29	28		
V_D/V_T	0.33	0.21		

IBW: ideal body weight

Reason for Stopping Test: (1) Groin pain; (2) leg pain; (3) dyspnea

Raw Data from Case 3 Exercise Test

Work (W)	$\dot{V}O_2$ (L/min)	$\dot{V}CO_2$ (L/min)	$\dot{V}E$ (L/min)	HR (bpm)	R	$\dot{V}E/\dot{V}O_2$	$\dot{V}E/\dot{V}CO_2$	$P_{ET}O_2$ (mmHg)	$P_{ET}CO_2$ (mmHg)
Rest	0.44	0.35	18	83	0.81	40	49	109	29
Unloaded	0.66	0.54	24	87	0.82	35	42	105	32
0	0.75	0.64	27	86	0.86	35	42	106	32
5	0.70	0.59	26	133	0.85	36	42	106	32
5	0.73	0.62	25	138	0.86	34	40	106	32
11	0.81	0.69	28	157	0.85	34	40	106	33
15	0.96	0.91	38	136	0.95	39	41	110	31
15	0.80	0.75	32	148	0.94	39	42	110	31
21	0.79	0.71	27	106	0.90	34	38	107	32
25	0.84	0.69	28	97	0.82	33	40	104	33
25	1.07	0.93	37	89	0.87	34	40	107	31
30	0.92	0.83	34	119	0.90	36	40	108	31
35	1.06	0.95	38	91	0.89	35	40	108	31
35	0.91	0.78	31	103	0.86	34	39	107	32
40	1.10	0.98	40	122	0.89	35	40	107	32
45	1.03	0.89	36	90	0.86	34	39	106	33
45	1.13	0.99	39	160	0.88	34	39	107	32
50	1.15	1.02	40	87	0.89	35	39	106	33
55	1.16	1.05	41	121	0.91	35	39	106	33
55	1.08	0.99	39	116	0.91	36	39	107	33
60	1.26	1.15	45	109	0.92	35	39	106	34
65	1.26	1.17	46	136	0.93	36	38	107	33
65	1.32	1.23	49	143	0.94	37	39	108	33
70	1.23	1.18	46	120	0.95	37	39	108	33
75	1.50	1.43	56	124	0.96	37	39	108	32
75	1.42	1.43	58	102	1.01	40	40	111	32
80	1.45	1.50	58	89	1.03	40	38	112	31
85	1.45	1.51	62	99	1.04	42	41	113	31
85	1.50	1.57	64	114	1.05	42	40	113	31
90	1.54	1.64	68	96	1.07	43	41	114	31
90	1.56	1.66	69	102	1.06	44	41	114	31
95	1.74	1.79	76	101	1.03	43	42	114	30
101	1.66	1.78	77	100	1.07	46	43	116	29
101	1.64	1.77	76	104	1.08	46	42	117	28
1-minute Recovery	1.204	1.473	62	103	1.22	51	42	119	30
5-minute Recovery	0.702	0.733	36	95	1.05	50	48	119	27

Self Assessment Case 3
9-Box Plot

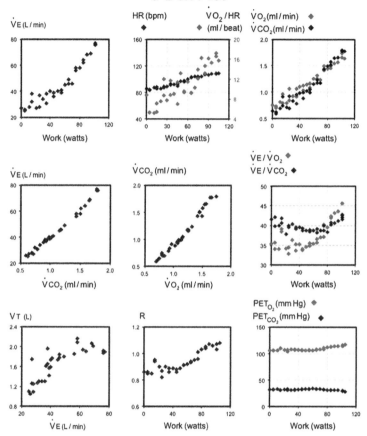

Fig. 7.3 Self-assessment case 3: 9-box plot

SELF-ASSESSMENT CASE 3: EXERCISE TEST INTERPRETATION WORKSHEET

Review the data from the test and provide your best assessment for each of the following variables:

		Pattern of limitation		
Observation	This patient	Cardiac	Pulmonary vascular/ILD	Ventilatory
Clear ventilatory threshold		•	•	
Plateau in O_2 pulse (end-exercise)		•	•	•[a]
High ($\dot{V}E / \dot{V}CO_2$) (mid-exercise)		•[b]	•	
High ($\dot{V}E / \dot{V}O_2$) (mid-exercise)		•[b]	•	
Large ventilatory reserve		•		
Metabolic acidosis by ABG (late exercise)		•	•	
Decreasing PETCO$_2$ (late exercise)		•	•	
R clearly rises above 1.0		•	•	
Stop exercising due to leg fatigue		•	•	
Heart rate near predicted maximum (late exercise)		•[c]		
ST changes on electrocardiography		•		
Inappropriate blood pressure response		•		
Increasing or unchanged VD/VT by ABG (late exercise)			•	
Absent ventilatory threshold				•
Decrease in oxygen saturation			•	•
Heart rate far below predicted maximum (late exercise)				•
Increasing or unchanged PETCO$_2$ (late exercise)				•
PaCO$_2$ ≥40 mmHg by ABG (end-exercise)				•
Small ventilatory reserve				•
Decreasing tidal volume				•
R does not increase above 1.0				•
Stop exercising due to dyspnea			•	•

[a] Can be seen when patients have severe air-trapping leading to increased intrathoracic pressure and decreased venous return

[b] High mid-exercise ventilatory equivalents for carbon dioxide and oxygen can be seen in severe cardiomyopathy. Many patients with cardiac limitation—including normal individuals and those with underlying cardiac disease—may still have normal ventilatory equivalents

[c] Not a reliable observation if the patient is on beta-blockers or has chronotropic limitation

Describe the $\dot{V}O_{2\,max}$:   Normal (>80% predicted): ____
                             Decreased (<80% predicted): ____

What do you think is the primary pattern of exercise limitation for this patient?

- Cardiac: ____
- Ventilatory: ____
- Pulmonary Vascular/Interstitial Lung Disease: ____

What testing or further evaluation should you pursue to follow up the results of this test?

SELF-ASSESSMENT CASE 4

Case Description: This is a 74-year-old man with a history of very severe COPD and mitral regurgitation who has been experiencing increasing dyspnea on exertion. The cardiologist has referred him for cardiopulmonary exercise testing to determine if he is more limited by his ventilatory impairment from COPD or from his valvular heart disease. The answer to this question will help determine whether he should be sent for further evaluation of his mitral valve issue and possible surgical repair.

Height: 179 cm

Weight: 88 kg

Pretest Pulmonary Function Tests:
FEV_1: 0.42 L (12% predicted)
FVC: 1.49 L (34% predicted)
FEV_1/FVC: 0.28
Maximum voluntary ventilation: 27 L/minute
Study performed while on supplemental oxygen (FIO_2 = 0.3)

Summary Data from Test:

Variable	Rest	Max	Predicted max	% Predicted
Work (W)	0	55	144	38
$\dot{V}O_2$ (ml/minute)	401	841	2,109	40
$\dot{V}O_2$ / kg (ml/kg/minute)	4.6	9.5	24.1	40
$\dot{V}O_2$ / kg IBW (ml/kg/minute)	4.6	9.5	24.1	40
Heart rate (bpm)	88	115	146	78.8
O_2 Pulse (ml O_2/beat)	5	8	14	55
Blood pressure (mmHg)	116/68	133/80		
Ventilation (L/minute)	15	29	27	110% of MVV
				173% of $FEV_1 \times 40$
Respiratory rate (bpm)	18	26		
Tidal volume (L)	0.83	1.22		
O_2 Saturation (%)	96	87		
$P_{ET}CO_2$ (mmHg)	41	50		

IBW: ideal body weight

Reason for Stopping Test: "I was running out of air"
Raw Data from Case 4 Exercise Test

Work (W)	$\dot{V}O_2$ (L/min)	$\dot{V}CO_2$ (L/min)	$\dot{V}E$ (L/min)	HR (bpm)	R	$\dot{V}E/\dot{V}O_2$	$\dot{V}E/\dot{V}CO_2$	$P_{ET}O_2$ (mmHg)	$P_{ET}CO_2$ (mmHg)
Rest	0.41	0.42	14.9	88	1.03	37	36	102	41
Unloaded	0.59	0.63	21.7	98	1.05	36	34	101	42
0	0.65	0.68	22.1	99	1.05	34	33	99	43
4	0.65	0.70	23.7	101	1.08	37	34	101	42
10	0.66	0.71	23.2	102	1.07	35	33	100	44
14	0.63	0.69	23.4	102	1.09	37	34	101	43
21	0.69	0.75	24.5	104	1.08	35	33	100	43
24	0.67	0.74	23.9	106	1.11	36	33	99	44
32	0.69	0.77	24.6	107	1.10	35	32	98	46
36	0.70	0.77	24.7	110	1.11	35	32	98	45
40	0.74	0.83	26.3	111	1.12	35	32	99	45
44	0.81	0.91	27.8	113	1.12	34	31	98	47
48	0.84	0.95	27.5	114	1.12	33	29	96	49
55	0.84	0.96	29.0	115	1.15	35	30	96	50
1-minute Recovery	0.84	1.06	30.1	115	1.20	34	28	97	49

Self Assessment Case 4
9-Box Plot

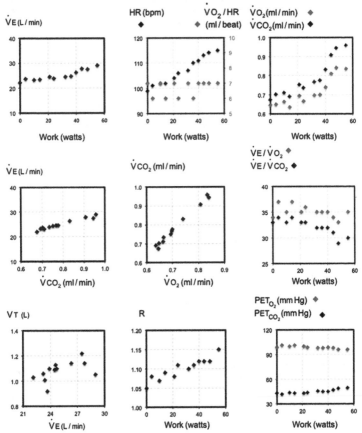

Fig. 7.4 Self-assessment case 4: 9-box plot

SELF-ASSESSMENT CASE 4: EXERCISE TEST INTERPRETATION WORKSHEET

Review the data from the test and provide your best assessment for each of the following variables:

| | | Pattern of limitation | | |
Observation	This patient	Cardiac	Pulmonary vascular/ILD	Ventilatory
Clear ventilatory threshold		•	•	
Plateau in O_2 pulse (end-exercise)		•	•	•[a]
High ($\dot{V}E / \dot{V}CO_2$) (mid-exercise)		•[b]	•	
High ($\dot{V}E / \dot{V}O_2$) (mid-exercise)		•[b]	•	
Large ventilatory reserve		•		
Metabolic acidosis by ABG (late exercise)		•	•	
Decreasing $PETCO_2$ (late exercise)		•	•	
R clearly rises above 1.0		•	•	
Stop exercising due to leg fatigue		•	•	
Heart rate near predicted maximum (late exercise)		•[c]		
ST changes on electrocardiography		•		
Inappropriate blood pressure response		•		
Increasing or unchanged VD/VT by ABG (late exercise)			•	
Absent ventilatory threshold				•
Decrease in oxygen saturation			•	•
Heart rate far below predicted maximum (late exercise)				•
Increasing or unchanged $PETCO_2$ (late exercise)				•
$PaCO_2$ ≥40 mmHg by ABG (end-exercise)				•
Small ventilatory reserve				•
Decreasing tidal volume				•
R does not increase above 1.0				•
Stop exercising due to dyspnea			•	•

[a] Can be seen when patients have severe air-trapping leading to increased intrathoracic pressure and decreased venous return

[b] High mid-exercise ventilatory equivalents for carbon dioxide and oxygen can be seen in severe cardiomyopathy. Many patients with cardiac limitation—including normal individuals and those with underlying cardiac disease—may still have normal ventilatory equivalents

[c] Not a reliable observation if the patient is on beta-blockers or has chronotropic limitation

Describe the $\dot{V}O_{2\,max}$:   Normal (>80% predicted): _____
                                    Decreased (<80% predicted): _____

What do you think is the primary pattern of exercise limitation for this patient?

- Cardiac: _____
- Ventilatory: _____
- Pulmonary Vascular/Interstitial Lung Disease: _____

What testing or further evaluation should you pursue to follow up the results of this test?

SELF-ASSESSMENT CASE 5

Case Description: 59-year-old man referred for cardiopulmonary exercise testing for evaluation of chronic cough and increasing dyspnea on exertion, the etiology of which remains unclear after an initial set of diagnostic studies.

Height: 185 cm

Weight: 92 kg

Pretest Pulmonary Function Tests:
FEV_1: 3.89 L (97% predicted)
FVC: 5.29 L (102% predicted)
FEV_1/FVC: 0.73 (predicted value 0.77)
TLC: 7.2 L (96% predicted)
DLCO: 21.4 ml/minute/mmHg (57% predicted)
Maximum voluntary ventilation: 172 L/minute

Summary Data from Test:

Variable	Rest	Max	Predicted max	% Predicted
Work (W)	0	183	193	95
$\dot{V}O_2$ (ml/minute)	454	2,116	2,896	73
$\dot{V}O_2$ / kg (ml/kg/minute)	4.9	22.9	37	62
$\dot{V}O_2$ / kg IBW (ml/kg/minute)	5.8	27	37	73
Heart rate (bpm)	82	167	161	104
O_2 Pulse (ml O_2/beat)	5.5	12.7	17	
Blood pressure (mmHg)	120/76	160/78		
Ventilation (L/minute)	17	117	172	68% of MVV
				75% of $FEV_1 \times 40$
Respiratory rate (bpm)	22	47		
Tidal volume (L)	0.80	2.34		
O_2 Saturation (%)	99	94		
$P_{ET}CO_2$ (mmHg)	32	25		

IBW: ideal body weight

ECG Results: No ST segment changes or arrhythmias noted.

Reason for Stopping Test: Dyspnea. He also became dizzy at the end of the test.

Raw Data from Case 5 Exercise Test

Work (W)	$\dot{V}O_2$ (L/min)	$\dot{V}CO_2$ (L/min)	$\dot{V}E$ (L/min)	HR (bpm)	R	$\dot{V}E/\dot{V}O_2$	$\dot{V}E/\dot{V}CO_2$	$P_{ET}O_2$ (mmHg)	$P_{ET}CO_2$ (mmHg)
Rest	0.45	0.38	17	79	0.84	37	44	115	32
Unloaded	0.78	0.64	26	88	0.82	33	40	114	33
2	0.74	0.70	27	91	0.95	36	38	117	33
7	0.74	0.67	25	92	0.90	33	37	115	33
12	0.85	0.74	30	87	0.87	34	39	115	33
16	0.82	0.74	29	94	0.91	34	38	117	32
22	0.85	0.78	28	92	0.91	32	36	116	33
28	0.79	0.73	28	93	0.92	35	37	117	32
33	0.88	0.79	29	96	0.90	33	36	115	33
38	0.97	0.86	32	100	0.89	32	36	116	33
43	0.98	0.90	34	98	0.91	34	37	116	33
47	1.01	0.93	34	102	0.92	33	36	116	33
52	1.01	0.94	34	106	0.93	33	35	116	34
56	1.12	1.04	37	109	0.93	33	35	116	33
61	1.15	1.09	39	112	0.94	33	35	116	33
66	1.14	1.10	38	114	0.97	33	34	117	33
71	1.19	1.13	40	118	0.95	33	35	116	33
75	1.34	1.29	46	118	0.96	34	35	118	32
79	1.25	1.22	45	122	0.98	35	36	118	33
84	1.35	1.33	48	121	0.98	35	35	118	32
88	1.41	1.40	49	125	1.00	34	35	118	33
92	1.46	1.48	52	128	1.01	35	35	120	32
97	1.51	1.58	58	132	1.05	38	36	121	31
100	1.55	1.63	59	134	1.05	38	36	122	31
105	1.47	1.58	56	137	1.08	38	35	122	31
109	1.58	1.67	58	142	1.05	36	35	121	31
114	1.64	1.78	63	144	1.08	38	35	123	30
118	1.59	1.73	61	145	1.09	38	35	123	31
122	1.71	1.88	68	146	1.10	39	36	123	30
126	1.69	1.88	66	147	1.11	39	35	124	30
130	1.75	1.95	70	150	1.12	39	35	124	30
133	1.75	1.99	72	151	1.13	41	36	125	29
137	1.80	2.05	75	153	1.14	41	36	125	29
140	1.84	2.05	73	153	1.12	39	35	123	30
144	1.89	2.14	78	154	1.14	41	36	124	30
148	1.92	2.14	74	155	1.11	38	34	123	31
151	2.07	2.39	92	156	1.16	44	38	126	28
154	1.95	2.27	86	158	1.17	43	37	126	29

Work (W)	$\dot{V}O_2$ (L/min)	$\dot{V}CO_2$ (L/min)	$\dot{V}E$ (L/min)	HR (bpm)	R	$\dot{V}E/\dot{V}O_2$	$\dot{V}E/ \dot{V}CO_2$	$P_{ET}O_2$ (mmHg)	$P_{ET}CO_2$ (mmHg)
157	2.10	2.49	99	160	1.18	47	39	128	27
160	2.05	2.45	98	162	1.20	47	39	128	27
163	2.10	2.55	105	163	1.22	50	41	129	26
165	2.06	2.51	102	165	1.22	49	40	128	27
168	2.14	2.57	106	167	1.20	49	41	129	26
171	2.14	2.56	108	167	1.20	50	42	129	26
173	2.21	2.71	115	165	1.22	51	42	130	25
176	2.12	2.61	109	167	1.23	51	41	130	25
178	2.23	2.69	117	167	1.20	52	43	130	25
181	2.14	2.60	114	167	1.22	53	43	130	25
183	2.16	2.60	111	167	1.21	51	42	130	25
1-minute Recovery	1.21	1.66	78	153	1.37	64	47	133	23
2-minute Recovery	1.02	1.32	64	136	1.3	62	48	131	25

Self Assessment Case 5
9-Box Plot

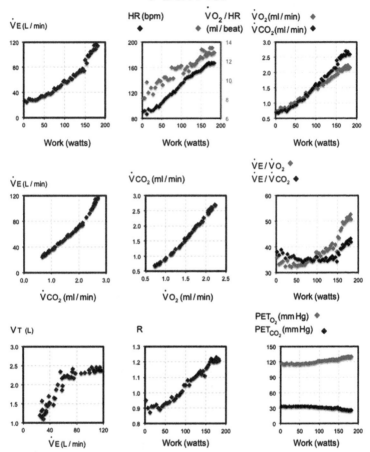

Fig. 7.5 Self-assessment case 5: 9-box plot

SELF-ASSESSMENT CASE 5: EXERCISE TEST INTERPRETATION WORKSHEET

Review the data from the test and provide your best assessment for each of the following variables:

Observation	This patient	Pattern of limitation		
		Cardiac	Pulmonary vascular/ILD	Ventilatory
Clear ventilatory threshold		•	•	
Plateau in O_2 pulse (end-exercise)		•	•	•[a]
High ($\dot{V}E / \dot{V}CO_2$) (mid-exercise)		•[b]	•	
High ($\dot{V}E / \dot{V}O_2$) (mid-exercise)		•[b]	•	
Large ventilatory reserve		•		
Metabolic acidosis by ABG (late exercise)		•	•	
Decreasing PETCO$_2$ (late exercise)		•	•	
R clearly rises above 1.0		•	•	
Stop exercising due to leg fatigue		•	•	
Heart rate near predicted maximum (late exercise)		•[c]		
ST changes on electrocardiography		•		
Inappropriate blood pressure response		•		
Increasing or unchanged VD/VT by ABG (late exercise)			•	
Absent ventilatory threshold				•
Decrease in oxygen saturation			•	•
Heart rate far below predicted maximum (late exercise)				•
Increasing or unchanged PETCO$_2$ (late exercise)				•
PaCO$_2$ ≥40 mmHg by ABG (end-exercise)				•
Small ventilatory reserve				•
Decreasing tidal volume				•
R does not increase above 1.0				•
Stop exercising due to dyspnea			•	•

[a] Can be seen when patients have severe air-trapping leading to increased intrathoracic pressure and decreased venous return

[b] High mid-exercise ventilatory equivalents for carbon dioxide and oxygen can be seen in severe cardiomyopathy. Many patients with cardiac limitation—including normal individuals and those with underlying cardiac disease—may still have normal ventilatory equivalents

[c] Not a reliable observation if the patient is on beta-blockers or has chronotropic limitation

Describe the $\dot{V}O_{2\,max}$:   Normal (>80% predicted): ____
                          Decreased (<80% predicted): ____

What do you think is the primary pattern of exercise limitation for this patient?
- Cardiac: ____
- Ventilatory: ____
- Pulmonary Vascular/Interstitial Lung Disease: ____

What testing or further evaluation should you pursue to follow up the results of this test?

ANSWERS TO SELF-ASSESSMENT CASES

ANSWERS TO SELF-ASSESSMENT CASE I

| | | Pattern of limitation | | |
| | This patient | Cardiac | Pulmonary vascular/ILD | Ventilatory |
Observation				
Clear ventilatory threshold	✓	•	•	
Plateau in O_2 pulse (end-exercise)	✓	•	•	•[a]
High ($\dot{V}E / \dot{V}CO_2$) (mid-exercise)		•[b]	•	
High ($\dot{V}E / \dot{V}O_2$) (mid-exercise)		•[b]	•	
Large ventilatory reserve		•		
Metabolic acidosis by ABG (late exercise)		•	•	
Decreasing $PETCO_2$ (late exercise)	✓	•	•	
R clearly rises above 1.0	✓	•	•	
Stop exercising due to leg fatigue		•	•	
Heart rate near predicted maximum (late exercise)	✓	•[c]		
ST changes on electrocardiography		•		
Inappropriate blood pressure response	✓	•		
Increasing or unchanged VD/VT by ABG (late exercise)			•	
Absent ventilatory threshold				•
Decrease in oxygen saturation			•	•
Heart rate far below predicted maximum (late exercise)				•
Increasing or unchanged $PETCO_2$ (late exercise)				•
$PaCO_2 \geq 40$ mmHg by ABG (end-exercise)				•
Small ventilatory reserve				•
Decreasing tidal volume				•
R does not increase above 1.0				•
Stop exercising due to dyspnea	✓		•	•

[a] Can be seen when patients have severe air-trapping leading to increased intrathoracic pressure and decreased venous return

[b] High mid-exercise ventilatory equivalents for carbon dioxide and oxygen can be seen in severe cardiomyopathy. Many patients with cardiac limitation—including normal individuals and those with underlying cardiac disease—may still have normal ventilatory equivalents

[c] Not a reliable observation if the patient is on beta-blockers or has chronotropic limitation

The $\dot{V}O_{2max}$ is decreased (<80% predicted)

Test Interpretation and Exercise Limitation Pattern

This patient demonstrates evidence of mild to moderately reduced exercise capacity. When adjusted for her actual body weight, her $\dot{V}O_{2\,max}$ of 25.3 ml/kg/minute represents 73% of predicted maximum. When normalized for her ideal body weight, her $\dot{V}O_{2\,max}$ of 28.8 ml/kg/minute represents 83% of her predicted maximum.

The data from the test indicate that she has a *cardiac pattern* as the source of her exercise limitation. She demonstrates evidence of a ventilatory threshold as demonstrated by several factors including the change in the slope of the relationship between $\dot{V}CO_2$ and $\dot{V}O_2$ (i.e., a change in her V-slope), the drop in her end-tidal carbon dioxide ($P_{ET}CO_2$) and rise in end-tidal oxygen ($P_{ET}O_2$) in late exercise, and the marked rise in her respiratory exchange ratio and ventilatory equivalents for oxygen and carbon dioxide ($\dot{V}E\,/\,\dot{V}O_2$ and $\dot{V}E\,/\,\dot{V}CO_2$) in late exercise. The ventilatory threshold is likely around 150 W and a $\dot{V}O_2$ of 1.5 L. The absence of oxygen desaturation in late exercise is also consistent with a cardiac source of exercise limitation as is her suboptimal blood pressure response. One atypical feature of her test, however, was that she stopped because of dyspnea. This is usually the reason for stopping in patients with ventilatory limitation, while patients with cardiac limitation usually stop because of leg fatigue. The fact that she was developing pre-syncopal symptoms at the end of the test and has a suboptimal blood pressure response, including a significant drop in her blood pressure after exercise was stopped, would fit with a cardiac etiology for her exercise limitation, however.

The patient does not demonstrate any evidence of ventilatory limitation. Although her minute ventilation at peak exercise approaches her maximum voluntary ventilation and $FEV_1 \times 40$ (slightly exceeding 80% of these values), she still has some ventilatory reserve and, more importantly, her $P_{ET}CO_2$ falls in late exercise. The change in $P_{ET}CO_2$ indicates that she is able to raise her minute ventilation in response to a developing metabolic acidosis. The presence of pre-syncope at end-exercise does raise concern about the possibility of pulmonary hypertension as the source of her symptoms but her mid-exercise ventilatory equivalents are lower than you would expect in this disorder and her dead-space fraction declines over the course of exercise. The latter finding is consistent with a cardiac limitation pattern and would not be seen in patients limited by pulmonary vascular disease.

What Testing or Further Evaluation Should You Pursue to Follow Up the Results of This Test?

The patient has a cardiac pattern of limitation and developed pre-syncopal symptoms at end-exercise that are very similar to what she develops when she exercises on her own. There are three possible causes for this clinical picture: myocardial ischemia, exercise-induced arrhythmia, or a stenotic valvular or other structural heart lesion limiting forward flow at peak exercise. Pulmonary hypertension should also be on the differential diagnosis for patients with exercise-associated syncope but in her particular case this is unlikely as her data are not consistent with a pulmonary vascular limitation since her dead-space fraction declined during her test. Her mid-exercise ventilatory equivalents for oxygen and carbon dioxide are also lower than you would expect in a patient with pulmonary hypertension.

The ECG in this study showed no evidence of ischemia and the patient did not develop any supraventricular or ventricular arrhythmias aside from her appropriate sinus tachycardia. This suggests that she may have a stenotic lesion limiting cardiac output at high levels of exercise, which can be further evaluated with an echocardiogram. The patient was subsequently sent for echocardiography and was found to have hypertrophic obstructive cardiomyopathy.

ANSWERS TO SELF-ASSESSMENT CASE 2

Observation	This patient	Pattern of limitation		
		Cardiac	Pulmonary vascular/ILD	Ventilatory
Clear ventilatory threshold	✓	•	•	
Plateau in O_2 pulse (end-exercise)	✓	•	•	•[a]
High ($\dot{V}E / \dot{V}CO_2$) (mid-exercise)	✓	•[b]	•	
High ($\dot{V}E / \dot{V}O_2$) (mid-exercise)	✓	•[b]	•	
Large ventilatory reserve	✓	•		
Metabolic acidosis by ABG (late exercise)	✓	•	•	
Decreasing $P_{ET}CO_2$ (late exercise)	✓	•	•	
R clearly rises above 1.0	✓	•	•	
Stop exercising due to leg fatigue	✓	•	•	
Heart rate near predicted maximum (late exercise)	✓	•[c]		
ST changes on electrocardiography		•		
Inappropriate blood pressure response		•		
Increasing or unchanged V_D/V_T by ABG (late exercise)	✓		•	
Absent ventilatory threshold				•
Decrease in oxygen saturation	✓		•	•
Heart rate far below predicted maximum (late exercise)				•
Increasing or unchanged $P_{ET}CO_2$ (late exercise)				•
$PaCO_2$ ≥40 mmHg by ABG (end-exercise)				•
Small ventilatory reserve				•
Decreasing tidal volume				•
R does not increase above 1.0				•
Stop exercising due to dyspnea	✓		•	•

[a] Can be seen when patients have severe air-trapping leading to increased intrathoracic pressure and decreased venous return

[b] High mid-exercise ventilatory equivalents for carbon dioxide and oxygen can be seen in severe cardiomyopathy. Many patients with cardiac limitation—including normal individuals and those with underlying cardiac disease—may still have normal ventilatory equivalents

[c] Not a reliable observation if the patient is on beta-blockers or has chronotropic limitation

The $\dot{V}O_{2max}$ is decreased (<80% predicted)

Test Interpretation and Exercise Limitation Pattern

This patient has evidence of significant exercise limitation. He achieves only 49% of his predicted work rate and, when adjusted for his actual body weight, his maximum oxygen uptake is only 55% of his predicted maximum.

The pattern of data is consistent with exercise limitation due to *pulmonary vascular* or *interstitial lung disease (ILD)*. There are several features of this case that are consistent with this finding. He has a high resting minute ventilation that could be due to a variety of factors, including possibly a high dead-space ventilation requirement. He has a ventilatory threshold as evidenced by the rise in his minute ventilation and $\dot{V}E / \dot{V}O_2$ and $\dot{V}E / \dot{V}CO_2$ as well as the decrease in $PETCO_2$ and $PaCO_2$ in late exercise (seen in both the numerical data and on the graphical displays). These changes are subtler than the changes in these parameters seen in Case 1, but they are present. The ventilatory threshold likely occurs around 65 W or a $\dot{V}O_2$ of 1.0 L. His oxygen saturation also falls during exercise from a baseline of 97 to 92%, a finding that would not be seen in cardiac limitation. Finally, and perhaps most important, his dead-space fraction (VD/VT) decreases only slightly from 0.48 at rest to 0.43 at peak exercise, a hallmark of the pulmonary vascular/interstitial lung disease pattern. Technically, the value did decline but a value this high at end-exercise is not normal. In patients with cardiac limitation, VD/VT should fall with increasing levels of work to significantly lower levels.

There is no evidence of ventilatory limitation as there is a large ventilatory reserve (peak minute ventilation 54% of MVV and 66% of $FEV_1 \times 40$) and $PETCO_2$ falls in late exercise. It should be noted that the $PaCO_2$ from the arterial blood gas is slightly higher at peak exercise than prior to exercise. This might make you think that ventilatory limitation is present. However, there are no blood gases from the middle of the exercise test to allow adequate assessment of the complete trend during the study. It is possible that the patient was hyperventilating in response to the ABG puncture before the exercise test giving a falsely low $PaCO_2$ at this time point.

What Testing or Further Evaluation Should You Pursue to Follow Up the Results of This Test?

The patient has a known form of interstitial lung disease, eosinophilic granuloma (pulmonary Langerhans histiocytosis). One of the mainstays of treatment for the disorder is smoking cessation, which the patient has not done. It is possible that the observed pattern on this test is due to worsening interstitial lung disease. This could be evaluated with a CT scan of the chest. As a complication of this and other forms of interstitial lung disease, however, patients can also develop pulmonary hypertension. As a result, it would be appropriate to also send this patient for an echocardiogram to measure his pulmonary arterial pressure.

ANSWERS TO SELF-ASSESSMENT CASE 3

		Pattern of limitation		
Observation	This patient	Cardiac	Pulmonary vascular/ILD	Ventilatory
Clear ventilatory threshold	✓	•	•	
Plateau in O_2 pulse (end-exercise)		•	•	•[a]
High ($\dot{V}E / \dot{V}CO_2$) (mid-exercise)	✓	•[b]	•	
High ($\dot{V}E / \dot{V}O_2$) (mid-exercise)	✓	•[b]	•	
Large ventilatory reserve		•		
Metabolic acidosis by ABG (late exercise)		•	•	
Decreasing PETCO$_2$ (late exercise)	✓	•	•	
R clearly rises above 1.0		•	•	
Stop exercising due to leg fatigue	✓	•	•	
Heart rate near predicted maximum (late exercise)		•[c]		
ST changes on electrocardiography		•		
Inappropriate blood pressure response	✓	•		
Increasing or unchanged VD/VT by ABG (late exercise)			•	
Absent ventilatory threshold				•
Decrease in oxygen saturation			•	•
Heart rate far below predicted maximum (late exercise)	✓			•
Increasing or unchanged PETCO$_2$ (late exercise)				•
PaCO$_2$ ≥40 mmHg by ABG (end-exercise)				•
Small ventilatory reserve	✓			•
Decreasing tidal volume				•
R does not increase above 1.0				•
Stop exercising due to dyspnea	✓		•	•

[a] Can be seen when patients have severe air-trapping leading to increased intrathoracic pressure and decreased venous return

[b] High mid-exercise ventilatory equivalents for carbon dioxide and oxygen can be seen in severe cardiomyopathy. Many patients with cardiac limitation—including normal individuals and those with underlying cardiac disease—may still have normal ventilatory equivalents

[c] Not a reliable observation if the patient is on beta-blockers or has chronotropic limitation

The $\dot{V}O_{2max}$ is decreased (<80% predicted)

Test Interpretation and Exercise Limitation Pattern

This patient demonstrates evidence of moderately reduced exercise capacity. When adjusted for his actual body weight, his $\dot{V}O_{2\,max}$ of 17.1 ml/kg/minute represents 52% of predicted maximum. When normalized for his ideal body weight, his $\dot{V}O_{2\,max}$ of 20.4 ml/kg/minute represents 62% of his predicted maximum.

The data from the test indicates that he has a *cardiac pattern* as the source of his exercise limitation. He demonstrates evidence of a ventilatory threshold as evidenced by several factors including the change in the slope of the relationship between $\dot{V}CO_2$ and $\dot{V}O_2$ (i.e., a change in his V-slope), the drop in his $PETCO_2$ and rise in $PETO_2$ in late exercise, and the rise in $\dot{V}E / \dot{V}O_2$ and $\dot{V}E / \dot{V}CO_2$ in late exercise. The ventilatory threshold is likely occurring around 60–65 W or a $\dot{V}O_2$ of 1.2–1.3 L. The patient's minute ventilation at peak exercise does rise to 89% of his MVV, a finding that is not common in cardiac limitation patterns except in highly fit athletes. This finding is suggestive of ventilatory limitation, but the other data (e.g., the drop in $PETCO_2$ at peak exercise, presence of a ventilatory threshold) all argue against ventilatory limitation as the source of his exercise limitation. The respiratory exchange ratio (R) does rise above 1.0 but does not rise as high as is often seen in patients with cardiac limitation.

In reviewing this patient's data, it is important to note that his heart rate is only 104 beats per minute at peak exercise compared to his age-predicted maximum of 145 beats per minute. He does have some higher heart rate values earlier in exercise but there is no steady rise in heart rate through the test and his heart rate is consistently lower at the end of the test than at the beginning. This suggests that the patient's cardiac limitation may be related to a *chronotropic problem* whereby the heart rate does not rise sufficiently in exercise to support an adequate cardiac output. Similar heart rate patterns can also be seen when patients are on beta-blocker therapy. The blood pressure also only rose to 125/70 at peak exercise, a suboptimal response that is often seen in patients with cardiomyopathy.

What Testing or Further Evaluation Should You Pursue to Follow Up the Results of This Test?

This patient should be referred to a cardiologist for further evaluation of his heart rate responses during exercise and whether or not he needs a pacemaker.

ANSWERS TO SELF-ASSESSMENT CASE 4

		Pattern of limitation		
Observation	This patient	Cardiac	Pulmonary vascular/ILD	Ventilatory
Clear ventilatory threshold		•	•	
Plateau in O_2 pulse (end-exercise)		•	•	•[a]
High ($\dot{V}E / \dot{V}CO_2$) (mid-exercise)		•[b]	•	
High ($\dot{V}E / \dot{V}O_2$) (mid-exercise)	✓	•[b]	•	
Large ventilatory reserve		•		
Metabolic acidosis by ABG (late exercise)		•	•	
Decreasing PETCO$_2$ (late exercise)		•	•	
R clearly rises above 1.0	✓	•	•	
Stop exercising due to leg fatigue		•	•	
Heart rate near predicted maximum (late exercise)		•[c]		
ST changes on electrocardiography		•		
Inappropriate blood pressure response		•		
Increasing or unchanged VD/VT by ABG (late exercise)			•	
Absent ventilatory threshold	✓			•
Decrease in oxygen saturation	✓		•	•
Heart rate far below predicted maximum (late exercise)	✓			•
Increasing or unchanged PETCO$_2$ (late exercise)	✓			•
PaCO$_2$ ≥40 mmHg by ABG (end-exercise)				•
Small ventilatory reserve	✓			•
Decreasing tidal volume				•
R does not increase above 1.0				•
Stop exercising due to dyspnea	✓		•	•

[a] Can be seen when patients have severe air-trapping leading to increased intrathoracic pressure and decreased venous return

[b] High mid-exercise ventilatory equivalents for carbon dioxide and oxygen can be seen in severe cardiomyopathy. Many patients with cardiac limitation—including normal individuals and those with underlying cardiac disease—may still have normal ventilatory equivalents

[c] Not a reliable observation if the patient is on beta-blockers or has chronotropic limitation

The $\dot{V}O_{2max}$ is decreased (<80% predicted)

Test Interpretation and Exercise Limitation Pattern

This patient has a very reduced maximum exercise capacity. When normalized for his actual and ideal body weights, his $\dot{V}O_{2\,max}$ of 9.5 ml/kg/minute represents only 40% of his predicted maximum.

The data in this case is consistent with a *ventilatory pattern* of exercise limitation. The patient's minute ventilation at peak exercise is 110% of his MVV and 173% of his $FEV_1 \times 40$. This indicates that he has no ventilatory reserve at end-exercise. In addition, his $PETCO_2$ rises throughout exercise, an important indication of ventilatory failure. Despite using supplemental oxygen, the patient also experiences a drop in his oxygen saturation during the test, a finding that can be seen in patients with either ventilatory or pulmonary vascular/ILD patterns of exercise limitation.

There is no evidence in this test that would fit with a cardiac pattern of limitation. He does not have a ventilatory threshold. His minute ventilation does not increase in late exercise, nor is there a change in the slope of the $\dot{V}CO_2$ vs. $\dot{V}O_2$ or $\dot{V}E$ vs. $\dot{V}CO_2$ relationships that is typically seen when the ventilatory threshold is reached. The $\dot{V}E / \dot{V}O_2$ and $\dot{V}E / \dot{V}CO_2$ also do not increase in late exercise. In fact, the $\dot{V}E / \dot{V}CO_2$ falls toward the end of the test as he goes into overt ventilatory failure and can no longer raise his minute ventilation in the face of increasing carbon dioxide production. His $\dot{V}E / \dot{V}O_2$ is mildly increased in mid-exercise, likely due to the fact that he has a high dead-space fraction, and does not increase in late exercise. Finally, he has a mildly increased heart rate reserve at end-exercise, as his heart rate reached only 78% of his age-predicted maximum.

What Testing or Further Evaluation Should You Pursue to Follow Up the Results of This Test?

This patient was sent for cardiopulmonary exercise testing to determine if his exercise capacity was limited by his COPD or by his valvular cardiomyopathy (mitral regurgitation). If it was determined that he had a cardiac limitation, it would have been reasonable to do further workup for mitral valve issue and consider a valve repair or replacement. However, because the data from this test show that he has ventilatory limitation as the primary source of limitation it would be appropriate to defer that workup and focus first on optimizing his COPD management. Were you to fix the mitral valve, he will likely be left with the same degree of exercise limitation from his severe COPD.

ANSWERS TO SELF-ASSESSMENT CASE 5

Observation	This patient	Cardiac	Pulmonary vascular/ILD	Ventilatory
Clear ventilatory threshold	✓	•	•	
Plateau in O_2 pulse (end-exercise)	✓	•	•	•[a]
High $(\dot{V}E / \dot{V}CO_2)$ (mid-exercise)	✓	•[b]	•	
High $(\dot{V}E / \dot{V}O_2)$ (mid-exercise)	✓	•[b]	•	
Large ventilatory reserve	✓	•		
Metabolic acidosis by ABG (late exercise)		•	•	
Decreasing $P_{ET}CO_2$ (late exercise)	✓	•	•	
R clearly rises above 1.0	✓	•	•	
Stop exercising due to leg fatigue		•	•	
Heart rate near predicted maximum (late exercise)	✓	•[c]		
ST changes on electrocardiography		•		
Inappropriate blood pressure response		•		
Increasing or unchanged V_D/V_T by ABG (late exercise)			•	
Absent ventilatory threshold				•
Decrease in oxygen saturation	✓		•	•
Heart rate far below predicted maximum (late exercise)				•
Increasing or unchanged $P_{ET}CO_2$ (late exercise)				•
$PaCO_2 \geq 40$ mmHg by ABG (end-exercise)				•
Small ventilatory reserve				•
Decreasing tidal volume				•
R does not increase above 1.0				•
Stop exercising due to dyspnea	✓		•	•

[a] Can be seen when patients have severe air-trapping leading to increased intrathoracic pressure and decreased venous return

[b] High mid-exercise ventilatory equivalents for carbon dioxide and oxygen can be seen in severe cardiomyopathy. Many patients with cardiac limitation—including normal individuals and those with underlying cardiac disease—may still have normal ventilatory equivalents

[c] Not a reliable observation if the patient is on beta-blockers or has chronotropic limitation

The $\dot{V}O_{2max}$ is decreased (<80% predicted)

Test Interpretation and Exercise Limitation Pattern

This patient demonstrates evidence of mild to moderately reduced exercise capacity. When adjusted for his actual body weight, his $\dot{V}O_{2\,max}$ of 22.9 ml/kg/minute represents 62% of predicted maximum. When normalized for ideal body weight, his $\dot{V}O_{2\,max}$ of 27 ml/kg/minute represents 73% of his predicted maximum.

The data from the test indicate that he has a *pulmonary vascular/ interstitial lung disease pattern* as the source of his exercise limitation. He demonstrates evidence of a ventilatory threshold as demonstrated by several factors including a drop in his end-tidal carbon dioxide ($P_{ET}CO_2$) and rise in end-tidal oxygen ($P_{ET}O_2$) in late exercise, as well as significant increases in the respiratory exchange ratio and ventilatory equivalents for oxygen and carbon dioxide ($\dot{V}E / \dot{V}O_2$ and $\dot{V}E / \dot{V}CO_2$) in late exercise. There is also a change in the slope of the relationship between $\dot{V}CO_2$ and $\dot{V}O_2$ (i.e., a change in his V-slope). The ventilatory threshold is likely around 100–110 W and a $\dot{V}O_2$ of 1.6 L.

While the presence of a clear ventilatory threshold is consistent with a cardiac pattern of limitation, there are two key findings that strongly suggest that the patient instead has a pulmonary vascular/ interstitial lung disease pattern. First, he demonstrated high ventilatory equivalents for both oxygen and carbon dioxide prior to the ventilatory threshold. Related to this is the fact that he also has a very high minute ventilation (16–18 L/minute at rest), which along with the high ventilatory equivalents, suggests that he likely has high physiologic dead space. The second distinguishing feature in this case is the fact that his oxygen saturation declined with increasing effort, a finding that is not seen in patients with cardiac limitation.

The case in favor of a pulmonary vascular/interstitial lung disease pattern of limitation could have been strengthened by measuring arterial blood gases during the test. In addition to confirming the presence of progressive impairment in oxygenation, blood gases would have permitted calculation of the dead-space fraction, a key variable for distinguishing between the cardiac and pulmonary vascular/interstitial lung disease patterns. As noted in Case 2 above and elsewhere in this primer, a stable or increasing dead-space fraction with progressive exercise is one of the physiologic hallmarks of the latter pattern.

From the data in the test alone, it is difficult to determine whether pulmonary vascular disease, such as pulmonary hypertension, or interstitial lung disease is responsible for his exercise limitation. One factor that is suggestive of interstitial lung disease is that his tidal volume plateaus at only about 44% of his vital capacity. As discussed in Chap. 3 (Fig. 3.6, Curve B in the bottom left graph) this is a lower level than that seen in normal individuals or patients with cardiac disease or isolated pulmonary vascular problems where the tidal volume usually plateaus at about two-thirds of the vital capacity.

Of note, the possibility of interstitial lung disease is not readily apparent on his pulmonary function testing, as is often the case in many patients with these disorders. Interstitial lung diseases typically cause a restrictive pattern on these tests in which you see reductions in the FEV_1 and FVC with a normal FEV_1/FVC ratio and, most importantly, a reduction in the total lung capacity (TLC, < 80% predicted). In this patient's case, however, the FEV_1, FVC, FEV_1/FVC, and TLC are all within the normal range predicted for someone of his age and height.

What Testing or Further Evaluation Should You Pursue to Follow Up the Results of This Test?

Because the data do not definitively distinguish between a pulmonary vascular process and interstitial lung disease, further testing is necessary to identify the primary problem. Echocardiography is warranted to evaluate the pulmonary artery pressure while a CT scan of the chest is indicated to assess for the presence of interstitial lung disease.

This patient underwent a CT scan, which demonstrated fibrotic changes in the peripheral regions of his basilar lung zones. He was subsequently sent for a surgical lung biopsy that revealed evidence of usual interstitial pneumonia, the histopathologic hallmark of the interstitial lung disease idiopathic pulmonary fibrosis.

About the Authors

Andrew M. Luks is an Associate Professor in the Department of Medicine (Division of Pulmonary and Critical Care Medicine) at the University of Washington.

Robb W. Glenny is a Professor in the Departments of Medicine and Physiology & Biophysics and serves as Head of the Division of Pulmonary and Critical Care Medicine at the University of Washington.

H. Thomas Robertson is Professor Emeritus in the Departments of Medicine (Division of Pulmonary and Critical Care Medicine) and Physiology & Biophysics at the University of Washington.

Index

A.M. Luks et al., *Introduction to Cardiopulmonary*
Exercise Testing, DOI 10.1007/978-1-4614-6283-5,
© Springer Science+Business Media New York 2013

Printed by Printforce, the Netherlands